Home and Away

Critical Perspectives on Psychology of Sexuality, Gender, and Queer Studies

Series Editors: A.L. Jones (Alice Miller School), Damien Riggs (Flinders University), and Rebecca Stringer (University of Otago)

Mission Statement

The series seeks to publish scholarship that engages critically with the social and political uses of psychological knowledge, and with transformative paradigms that address obstacles to change. The series is open to a wide range of approaches that may be classified as "psychological," including manuscript proposals that focus on well-being, subjectivities, clinical practice, discourse, and their intersections.

Books in Series

Home and Away: Mothers and Babies in Institutional Spaces, by Kathleen Connellan, Clemence Due, Damien W. Riggs, and Clare Bartholomaeus

Assisted Reproduction: Conceptions, Controversies, and Community Sentiment, by Alexandra Sigillo and Monica Miller

The Reproductive Industry: Intimate Experiences and Global Processes, edited by Vera Mackie, Nicola J. Marks, and Sarah Ferber

The Psychic Life of Racism in Gay Men's Communities, edited by Damien Riggs

Home and Away

Mothers and Babies in Institutional Spaces

Kathleen Connellan, Clemence Due,
Damien W. Riggs, and Clare Bartholomaeus

LEXINGTON BOOKS
Lanham • Boulder • New York • London

Published by Lexington Books
An imprint of The Rowman & Littlefield Publishing Group, Inc.
4501 Forbes Boulevard, Suite 200, Lanham, Maryland 20706
www.rowman.com

6 Tinworth Street, London SE11 5AL, United Kingdom

British Library Cataloguing in Publication Information Available

Library of Congress Cataloging-in-Publication Data

Names: Connellan, Kathleen Anne, 1959- author.
Title: Home and away : mothers and babies in institutional spaces / Kathleen Connellan, Clemence Due, Damien W. Riggs, Clare Bartholomaeus.
Description: Lanham : Lexington Books, [2020] | Series: Critical perspectives on the psychology of sexuality, gender, and queer studies | Includes bibliographical references and index. | Summary: "Home and Away provides a comprehensive account of critical design for mental health, focusing on how health facilities can intentionally promote positive psychological outcomes through design and use of space"— Provided by publisher.
Identifiers: LCCN 2020033148 (print) | LCCN 2020033149 (ebook) | ISBN 9781498592918 (cloth) | ISBN 9781498592925 (epub) Subjects: LCSH:
Mothers—Mental health services. | Mothers—Institutional care. | Mental health facilities. | Interior decoration—Psychological aspects. | Maternal health services.
Classification: LCC RC451.4.W6 C6725 2020 (print) | LCC RC451.4.W6 (ebook) | DDC 362.2082—dc23
LC record available at https://lccn.loc.gov/2020033148
LC ebook record available at https://lccn.loc.gov/2020033149-4985-9291-8

Contents

List of Figures

Acknowledgments

We acknowledge that we live and work on the land of the Kaurna people, and we acknowledge their sovereignty as First Nations people.

We thank the staff at Lexington Books, Kasey Beduhn and Julie Kirsch, for their assistance and support, as well as the series editors, Rebecca Stringer and Al Jones for supporting the inclusion of the book in the series. We also thank audiences of the Australasian Marcé Society for Perinatal Mental Health 2015 conference, the Australian Psychological Society College of Health Psychologists 2015 conference, and the Fay Gale Centre 2015 conference for feedback on project findings. We are grateful to the clinicians and staff in the mother-baby unit where the research was conducted for their time and enthusiasm in ensuring the smooth operation of our work on site. We thank the mothers staying in the unit and their families for allowing us to visit. We are also most appreciative to the architects for sharing information so that their work could be evaluated and to Roxanne Adams who assisted with architectural data. Special thanks go to Maddie Schiller for the cover drawing. Finally we acknowledge the University of South Australia for the Divisional Research Performance Fund grant.

Chapter 1

Introduction

> *I have been in other psych wards,—I hated them*, I felt trapped. 'Cos I was in the B Ward [psychiatric ward] as a teenager and it's very much—just it looks like a hospital [laughs uncomfortably] it looks like a hospital room, the lights are all orangey yellow and the walls are all pasty yellowish white and the lounge room looks like a hospital lounge room and the bedrooms look like hospital rooms. This feels more like a hotel [laughs] really (emphasis added).

The extract above is taken from an interview with a mother in the state-run psychiatric mother-baby unit (MBU) that provides the data for this book. This mother emphasizes the difference between feeling "trapped" in badly lit yellowed spaces in a psychiatric ward and feeling like she is in a "hotel" in an MBU. From her words, going to a hotel is perhaps a bit special, maybe even a privilege. This is a young woman who has been in and out of mental health units and is now struggling with a new child. Therefore, and perhaps for the first time, the space itself helps to build her self-worth. There is no doubt that dingy buildings are depressing, but how can new designs really make a difference? This is something we continue to ask. A fresh opportunity to research a recent design of an MBU in a larger repurposed mental health facility offered more questions and perhaps some answers. These are explored and discussed in the chapters that follow.

Women's placement into asylums and similar institutions simply for showing their feelings was common particularly in the seventeenth, eighteenth, and nineteenth centuries in Europe. When this occurred women who were mothers were always separated from their children. Patriarchal norms weakened in the twentieth century as more women entered the field of psychiatry. Mental health facilities began to be acknowledged as places that can intentionally promote positive psychological outcomes for both mothers and their children through the design of the facility and the use of space. A departure from the asylum-style to one that sought to simulate a domestic environment dovetailed changes in models of care which also became more human centered. Concomitant changes occurred in relation to psychiatric care for mothers and the practice of keeping them with their infants, rather than separating mothers and babies, led to the inception of purpose built psychiatric MBUs. Today MBUs that keep the child with the mother are regarded as best practice in many countries (Royal Australian & New Zealand College of Psychiatrists 2015). MBUs are separated from other adult mental health facilities and provide therapeutic accommodation as well as crucial clinical support for the mother and baby. MBUs are discrete units available to mothers who experience significant mental health conditions in the postpartum period. A background to MBUs is detailed in chapter 2 "An Overview of Psychiatric Mother-Baby Unit Research."

This book intersects the fields of psychology, psychiatry, nursing, occupational therapy, and health, with those of architecture, interior design, and gender studies. In order to serve a diverse readership, our approach brings together a broad range of human and design perspectives to contribute to the evidence base for critical mental health design. The title *Home and Away: Mothers and Babies in Institutional Spaces* encapsulates these crossovers where vulnerable psychologies and fragile bodies occupy a singular designed space to shape damaged maternal and familial relationships. This first chapter sets the conceptual framework by introducing the reader to the intersecting fields of gender, space, and health, before moving on to privacy and regulation, which includes a focus on space and movement. A discussion of terminology, subject positioning, and language follows so that the theoretical and methodological framework of the book is clear. We argue that a multidisciplinary approach is essential to understanding the differences across staff hierarchies, client uniqueness, and architectural vision, and suggest that, to date, gender has been largely overlooked in discussions of design for mental health.

The concept of home for a diverse group of mothers, babies, families, and staff is continually questioned in this book and underpins our approach. Crucially, the book shows that while mothers in institutional care are away from their own homes, they are not away from their babies; therefore, we analyze the way that mothers respond to the space and the way that the space responds to their needs for privacy, rest, routine, and wellness in a way that simulates home. The role of staff in a space that is ambiguously homely and clinical adds a dimension to our enquiry into the effectiveness of the domestic/work balance. Additionally, the inclusion of family members as visitors or co-residents with their partners or daughters adds a layer to the success of the designed spaces. The book seeks to answer four key research questions: (1) How can built space affect the relationships and interaction between staff and clients? (2) How can built space affect the work and well-being of staff? (3) How can built space affect interactions between clients and their families? and (4) How can built space impact on clients, staff, and families in terms of gender and other aspects of identity (e.g., culture or age)? A central aim of the book is to show how the structural and ambient design of MBUs shapes the experiences of those who occupy it. These occupants (mothers, babies, families, and a range of clinical and support staff) are predominantly women.

This book considers the processes involved in designing the facilities and the use of space in purpose built MBUs. To do this, the book draws on a comprehensive case study of an MBU in Australia to explore the practical outcomes of critical mental health design. The case study brings together interviews with key stakeholders (architects, staff, and clients) and an ethnography conducted by the authors to explore how a purpose built space for mental health works in practice. Importantly, this multifaceted strategy allows for an overarching consideration of the design, the designers, and the users of the space. This includes the architects' understandings of design for perinatal mental health and approaches for communicating and consulting with health department administrators and clinicians. Additionally, a multivalent technique helps to expose how spaces actually work in practice, drawing on researcher observations, and views of staff and clients which in turn are compared to visions of the architects. The different data sets as well as the multidisciplinary research team inform how the spaces imitate a domestic milieu for mothers, babies, and their families, and how this is gendered. Furthermore, the varied expertise allows for a broader contextual analysis of where purpose built designs work as therapeutic spaces and where they do not. Staff views of how spaces function as workspaces and how this impacts on their well-being as well as facilitates interpersonal relationships between staff and clients is an important addition to the overall analysis. Finally, the clients' own views of how purpose built designs work as therapeutic spaces for them is of immense importance. Throughout the book, the case study will be situated within the broader literature context, in relation to both mental health design and the historical context of women and mental health facilities.

There is an increasing recognition of the importance of design on mental health, yet little empirical research has been conducted into how the design of a facility itself shapes the experiences of those who occupy it. We offer in-depth empirical research on critical design for the mental health of mothers and babies. In the process we provide a critique of current consultation and evaluation practices and we recommend specific improvements. The focus on case study material means the points in the book are clear and accessible to a wide range of audiences and we hope to satisfy the needs of academics and researchers, particularly those working in the areas of health design, mental health/psychology, mental health nursing, sociology of health/illness, and gender studies.

It is also our intention to ensure that this text is accessible to primary healthcare professionals, particularly in mental health, including psychologists, psychiatrists, mental health nurses, and occupational therapists. This reach extends to policymakers in health, and finally to architects and interior designers working in mental health building design. We also focus on critical health design so that practical findings and applications of the research can be useful for mental health professionals working in a range of areas. Specifically, we highlight which aspects of design promote well-being, alongside a focus on potential barriers arising from design aspects. A background of the current contexts of mental health facilities is provided, as well as the ways in which space can be best designed for positive mental health outcomes. As mentioned above, this includes an emphasis on the importance of improved consultation processes, pre- and post occupancy evaluations, and their role in further improving future purpose built facilities. Important information is provided on the need for comprehensive contextualized consultation processes involved in designing purpose built facilities that should ensure the principles of health design are paired with achieving positive mental health outcomes. Therefore, in many ways the book is directly relevant to architects and interior designers working in health building design, offering perspectives of architects involved in this work, as well as an in-depth consideration of how designs function in practice.

Design for health and mental health in particular is a growing field and its expanse is perhaps also its problem. There is a need to think small and not big, to put the person at the center rather than a grand vision. The person in this instance is the mother, her child, her partner, and her clinicians; all move and operate in the apparent solidity of an MBU. Our critical appraisal of health design deliberately "disturbs and fragments, it reveals the fragility of that which seems solid" (Rose 1998, 41). Light, air, sounds, smells, and views all permeate the boundaries of architectural space to affect the therapeutic milieu and affordances of the building.

The literature on health design and the benefits of obvious things like natural light, fresh air, a view of nature and access to nature, privacy, and quiet have attracted many studies (Connellan et al. 2013). The redesign and new builds of psychiatric hospitals is ongoing, with a move away from large landscaped grounds to more compactly designed spaces, frequently reassigning premises and precincts for urban housing development (Wood et al. 2015). The unit that is the focus of our study is just such an example. The lands of the old asylum styled buildings, while previously on the edges of the city, are now prime real estate. The challenge was to meet the demands of developers and state health authorities as the old buildings and extensive grounds were proposed for redistribution and development. There is no question that asylums fell short of being therapeutic spaces but what many did have in their favor were vast grounds and gardens with established trees and lawns (Hickman 2009). The loss of a natural setting in contemporary psychiatric design should not necessarily mean neglecting essential healing aspects of natural light and fresh air. However, design technologies, security precautions, and climate conditions are not always in sync with healing. The inequalities of all these aspects interlock in spatial relations of gender and health, concepts that frame the approach of this book (Massey 1994).

CONCEPTUAL FRAMING: GENDER, SPACE, AND HEALTH

There is plenty about sex but little about gender in the histories of mental health. Michel Foucault (1978) in *The History of Sexuality* notes that sexual deviances, obsessions, and other aspects within its discourse multiplied themselves in a misunderstood milieu of morality. Foucault observes that all these discussions were too readily pathologized and held under a shroud of silence in ordinary society. Even though Sigmund Freud (2010) appeared to lift the taboos on writing openly about sex in the late nineteenth and early twentieth century, he also contributed to binary separations of male and female. The hierarchy of "culture" (male) above "nature" (female) was closely associated with biological difference. These divisions, at least in the west, stretch as far back as Plato (1935), writing more than 300 years BC, who in his *Republic* transcribes Socrates's debate on the role and place of women.

Today, both gender and sexuality eschew biological determinism, and understanding of sex as socially constructed is promoted by feminists who claim the social agency of diverse bodies (Kelly 2016). Nonetheless, gender prejudices remain in some spheres (Scott 2000; Torgrimson and Minson 2005). Residual fears of unconventional approaches to medicine once viewed as women's witchcraft recall a time when, if women were not "good" mothers and wives, they were mad (Kelly 2016). Under systemic patriarchies, female "conditions" were largely associated with hysteria and an inability to perform firmly circumscribed female duties (McClintock 1995; Oakley 1974; Tasca et al. 2012). As such, women were always already regarded as unstable. Foucault's *History of Madness* (2006) has substantial entries for women and madness. There was a gendering of madness that assigned nervous conditions, and hysteria in particular, to women.

While the account above may all sound historic, such prejudice lies in the wings of twenty-first-century mental health wards; gender definitely matters, with women in the mental health system still seen as more "difficult" than men (Bartlett and Somers 2017). Annie Bartlett and Nadia Somers's work shows that women are regarded as more emotionally demanding than men and staff in women's mental health wards suffer more burnout than in men's wards (Bartlett and Somers 2017). It is likely that staff fatigue in women's wards may in turn perpetuate perceptions that women are more demanding than men in mental health wards. Foucault (2006) points out that hysteria was a "catch-all" for the ignorance of doctors in the eighteenth and nineteenth centuries. Such perceptions of hysteria included an "internal heat that spread throughout the body . . . thought to be similar to the amorous ardour with which hysteria is often linked, as in young women seeking a match or young widows who had lost their husbands" (Foucault 2006, 280). This image is attributed to Jacques Ferrand in his seventeenth-century *Maladie d'amour ou mélancolie érotique*. Within such conjured images of instability, sex is repeatedly the critical point upon and around which diagnoses were based. As such women were not gendered but sexed in a way that connected them to animals (Foucault 2006).

In the twentieth and twenty-first centuries feminists have turned previous uneasiness of sex, nature, and power around. Elizabeth Grosz (2005) and Luce Irigaray (1991) reclaim biological aspects of women as enabling rather than limiting. This move also disturbs nature/culture hierarchies in the sense that nature is productive of culture and not inhibiting (Grosz 2005). Understanding the productive powers of what is deemed to be "natural" in everyone is vital not only for gender, sexuality, and queer studies but also for architectural designs. To codify "woman" is reductive and damaging (Scott 2000). Later in this chapter, the intricacies of language and subjectivities are discussed, but firstly dynamics between sex, nature, and gender as they move into and build culture require more discussion. On these grounds and specifically in the context of this book it is women who give birth to babies, a "natural" event that collides with culture.

Grosz (2005, 45) writes that "[c]ulture scripts the natural; it writes it, divides it, manufactures it in socially useful, palatable, and expected forms." Capitalist society has reconstructed the "natural," and cultural stereotypes risk becoming the "natural." In this way the mother of a child is assigned roles and places in a culture still complicated by gender struggles. Gendered roles of woman as mother, wife, carer, cook, and cleaner have not disappeared. Expectations that at least some, if not all, of the above are duties may not be uttered out loud, but familial and community connections unwittingly perpetuate the idea. These "duties" have been domesticated into a cult over time with women at the center. The cult of domesticity creates an aura of home as sacred and a space that is protected (Connellan 2016). As with all cults, control and secrecy operate behind its façade of peace, order, and harmony.

The myth of perfect children, a perfect home, and a good mother is dangerous and can easily lead to mental and physical breakdown. Society perpetuates false ideas of home life and unrealistic standards that contribute to mothers' perinatal ill health. It may no longer be the 1950s when the domestic appliance "revolution" flooded society with media images of happy housewives, smiling children, and shiny kitchens, but the myth lingers (Connellan 2016).

Home is therefore both a symbolic and a material space. The spaces that are shaped as home, the people called family, and the objects that inhabit those relational spaces can be very easily ruptured (Connellan 2018). There is an intertextual relationship between individuals and their personal spaces and belongings that can either help or hinder their well-being (Miller 2001). Maternal practices operate "through engagements with the non-human" (Boyer 2018, 3). The spatial and material design of a home provides a subjectifying framework with "motherhood [as] a spatial practice," and while the home-space is crucial, mothering does not stop there (Boyer 2018, 3). The MBU that is the focus of this book, which we have chosen to call "Park House," attempts to create an aura of "home" for the practices of motherhood. It is a formidable task because it can never be home, so it tries at the very least not to be a hospital space that speaks of sickness (Chrysikou 2014). In an MBU the spaces are functional and not personal and the objects within them represent a group rather than individuals. A home-space that is also a health-space unavoidably presents the ruptures that brings the mothers and babies into its enclosure, despite Park House's attempts to hide the clinical language of the space.

The specific needs of women in psychiatric units require more attention not only in terms of their admission characteristics, care pathways, and background health issues, but also with regard to the physical design and precinct of the unit (Archer, Lau, and Sethi 2016). The importance of close collaboration with architects, clinicians, and the occupiers of the newly designed psychiatric spaces is acknowledged but rarely implemented well (Long et al. 2011). In this book, it is not only the mothers and clinicians in the unit that are of interest, but the gender of the chief designers and the decision makers that resulted in the new build. Design for health does not begin with the first brick but rather with the first idea. Ideas can be borne out of dreams, mistakes, and experience, but they then need to be shared, agreed upon, and budgeted for. All of these processes involve design thinking and a meeting of different minds and bodies, which can often be the problem. Design thinking, architecture, mental health, and perinatal mental health are all gendered in some way. All too often health design thinking is just that: it is thinking and not feeling, and it forgets the embodied experience of the internal spaces. Mental health does not only reside in the head but in the entire body. Therefore, design for mental health and specifically for perinatal mental health cannot be compartmentalized; it must of necessity consider bodies and relationships. In this vein, there is a need for a feminist sociology of health care design, alongside the already extensive work of feminist geographers (Martin et al. 2015).

The link between mother, baby, gender, and home can be seen as part of a troubled symbolic order in gender, space, and interior architecture. Diane Agrest (2000) provides a reminder of the historic logocentric connection between the male body and western architecture. The Vitruvian male body with outstretched legs and arms, forming a perfect circle in a square was used for centuries as the standard measure for architectural design: it is the classical trope of form and function reinforced in modernist architecture (Connellan 2010a, 2013; Pevsner 1975). Interestingly, Penny Sparke (2008) asserts that the traditional architectural separations of the exterior (male) public sphere and interior (female) private sphere ran into problems when the exterior and interior became increasingly merged in open-plan modernist designs. Sparke notes that some male architects' solution to this was to "eliminate the interior by subordinating it to [male] architecture" (2008, vii). Agrest (2000) goes further than this citing that the conception and birth of a new building became the male architect's way of subsuming the female gender. These seemingly radical inversions of gender and architecture are complex and often only implicit; our study highlights the instability of the masculine logocentric order in MBU architecture.

When the authors of this book published a literature review article on mental health and architectural design, the state of the research showed a lack of evidence-based studies (Connellan et al. 2013; Urbanoski 2013). This remains the case but, as is discussed in chapter 2 of this book, there is also a need for more nuanced qualitative research into the importance of gender in the architectural design of women's mental health facilities. While there is research on architecture, gender, and health, there is no substantial evidence of what women's needs might be. It is agreed that gender matters, but insufficient specifics are at hand (Biancheri and Landi 2016). Many universities have now established research centers to promote and attract funding for studies across mental health and design, but to date there is limited research on design for mothers and babies in the perinatal period as the literature review in chapter 2 shows.

The "psy" disciplines, which include psychology, psychotherapy, psychoanalysis, and psychiatry, together form an "intellectual technology" and jointly provide methods of forming and understanding the self (Rose 1998, 11). A subject that is dealt with in more detail later in this chapter, and also in the data chapters, is that these surveillance technologies which govern parenthood, children, and family life only increase their difficulties (Rose 1999).

Parents, and mothers in particular, who crack under the pressure of the mythological demands of a "good" home and a "good" mother are frequently disenfranchised through lack of access to social support. This is partially the fault of neoliberalism and the rebounding effects of biopolitics (Foucault 2008). Expectations of parenting performance have become part of a much larger economy. Relationships are inverted from the social to the economic (Foucault 2008). Buildings and services are funded, designed, built, and staffed all in the name of social development. Clinics, counseling centers (both inside and outside of hospitals), and schools make up the fabric of large administrative and organizational controls. Rose (1999, viii) writes that these forms of regulation "do not crush subjectivity [but] actually fabricate subjects." It is possible that in a triad of power, knowledge, and subjectivity, individual realities are sacrificed in favor of in a larger scheme that labels motherhood, parenthood, and childhood as firmly understood and shared concepts.

There is a crucial and even defining element of an ideal home that an MBU tries to ensure, and that is safety. Home as a place of safety is something that people live and die for (Connellan 2018). Security and privacy is a cherished concept in the intimacies of motherhood, but when that safety is under threat then a mother and her child may move to an MBU for assistance. Women who seek help in this way want to be listened to respectfully and to be safe, and unfortunately a hospital setting is not always a place of safety for women (Copperman and Knowles 2006).

PRIVACY AND REGULATION

Ways that both freedom and privacy operate within the controls of an MBU is contingent on the differing realities and identities of individual mothers. Most of the mothers admitted to MBUs are there out of choice and clinical recommendation, and therefore we do not focus specifically on mothers who were sectioned in this book. In our case study, only two mothers were on mental health order during our observations and for the majority of mothers the therapeutic treatment is one of freedom and not coercion (Rose 1998). Nonetheless, there is a distinct overlap here between subjectivation and freedom. Freedom to be safe and to feel hope for the future is at the heart of a therapeutic milieu. Drawing from Foucault's lectures *On the Government of the Living*, if a person seeks internal direction, the "formula" is: "I freely obey what you will for me," in this way, there is a relinquishing of freedom based on trust (Foucault 2012, 231). At the same time, there remains a certain and crucial obligation to be "free" to learn and to adjust one's behavior or type of mothering (Rose 1998, 78). Therefore, there are layers of freedom and these are made manifest by the ability to leave the MBU building and go for a walk, knowing that it is a small freedom within a larger framework of governing of the self and others (Foucault 2010; Rose 1998). Consequently, it is a case of "you are free to be free" *but* there are conditions (Foucault 2008). These conditions are not only set out in the mothers' separate care plans, but they are also laid out materially in the arrangement of the built spaces. In such an atmosphere of being free and simultaneously monitored, there must be somewhere the mothers can go and be alone, out of sight and sound, somewhere to just be. But in an MBU there is not; while there are no cameras in the bedrooms, sounds are recorded to alert the nurses of crying babies.

In this way privacy raises its head as an important consideration. Privacy, in a new era of person-centered mental health, is also a respect for others' privacy. For example, the nurses' respect for the mothers is important here, as is the architects' understanding of this crucial aspect in the design of the unit. Then there is the researcher conducting ethnographic observation: the researcher who sits, watches, and takes notes, trying to be as unobtrusive as possible. Therefore, privacy affects all users of the MBU; it is not only privacy for the mothers but also for the nurses who spend long hours in a reciprocal type of surveillance. The nurses see and hear, and are in turn seen and heard. There is a whole system of visualization in an MBU that is not immediately as obvious as it might be in, for example, an acute adult mental health unit where the nurses' station still operates as a panopticon and lines of sight are unimpeded (Due, Connellan, and Riggs 2012). These techniques of visualization in the MBU render the visibilities and invisibilities as less obvious (Rose 1998, 1999). Consequently, there is more potency in the *hidden* grid of architectural design that operates in tandem with models of care in an MBU (Connellan et al. 2013). Additionally, babies and toddlers are subjected to the panoptic gaze in what Rose calls the "child panopticon" (1999, 146).

In a semblance of democratic design where users have equal agency in the spaces, all is not what it seems. Architectural design for mental health entered the postmodern era of ostensible inclusiveness with light, free flowing spaces decades ago. This means there are fewer sequestered spaces and less privacy, but the ubiquitous openness allows for constant surveillance in the guise of freedom. There was a move away from the obvious hierarchies of hospital wards and corridors apparent in both nineteenth-century asylum design and twentieth-century modernism. This shift takes on a "new *democratic* legitimacy" while maintaining careful regulation of functional spaces for clinical practice based on established knowledge (Rose 1998, 90). The ability for architectural design to prescribe activities and movements in and through space is particularly potent in institutions, including MBUs, which is a focus of this book (Gillespie 2002).

The divide between public and private spheres is more marked in a home outside of an institution where there may be a garden wall and gate or a secured entrance to an apartment. In that context, there are laws against trespassing those thresholds, but also social mores surrounding visiting another's home. In an MBU, the public and private spheres are not as distinct and the rules are different. Mothers and their families are conscious of being observed. Confidentiality and conversation come into focus in open-plan spatial design where even spontaneity is designed. In the client interview data, one mother said that she felt more comfortable developing her relationship with her baby privately than in the communal room. Another client said that, despite the openness, she felt everything was stuck together and that she was constantly watched. The expectation to be "natural" and relaxed just because the open-plan design allows for this is not a simple translation from built space to psychic space. If conversation requires privacy, a physical move to a counseling room may be necessary, but is not always possible. In this way balances between clinical confidentiality and conversational openness are constantly at play.

One mother's reality is not another's and this diversity extends to the spaces they inhabit and use for mothering. "In lay terms the real is the here and now" (Connellan 2019), but even this is a contested zone. For example, for Lacan (2006) the real is primal and deep. Nonetheless, realities in design are often conceived as "truths" from a functional point of view. For example, "this is the lounge" where you relax and take time out with your baby just as "this is the nursery" where the baby sleeps. The reality of what happens in those spaces may be far from ascribed truths of relaxation, play, or sleep. All of the spaces in an MBU cannot always replicate realities of home; the very idea of home has multiple kinds of "truth" and "is not just one place" (Massey 1994, 171). An MBU as an "institution" is itself a kind of "truth." The organization of an MBU such as Park House is a "bounded and administered space, an architectural form and an enclosure for powers and hierarchies, [it] produces new conditions for knowing individuals and problematizes new questions concerning their management" (Rose 1998, 122). We are most interested in the new questions that arise from mothers and staff in an MBU; expectations of an "ideal" family or mother are never simple. As stated earlier, realities are multiple and dynamic, and despite the "polyvalent counter-discourse that sought to 'restore' the family its 'rights' to autonomy and privacy . . . the modern private family remains intensively governed" (Rose 1999, 212).

An MBU may not have the gender separation that still exists in families and homes in the twenty-first century, but it may inadvertently reinforce the burden of child caring as a woman's role. It is, after all, an MBU full of women who are mothers. It is particularly significant that Park House permits partners of the mother to stay with the mother in a "family bedroom." There may be an assumption in an MBU that all partners of the mothers are men and this is certainly something that remains open for future research. Nonetheless, the absence of apparent gendered tasks and gendered spaces in an MBU may indeed be very different to some of the mothers' actual experience when at home with their partner and babies. There may be an artificial or unrealistic semblance of a gender neutral home environment in an MBU, where particular mothers' realities are far removed from such equalities. Outside of an MBU realities of family life are masked (Rose 1998), but the expectation within the boundaries of the MBU is that both fantasies and actualities are faced as part of what may still be situated within a "psychiatric truth" (Foucault 2003). In line with postmodernism, Foucault (2003, 2011, 2017) unravels multiple "truths" and decries the universality of "truth." He shows how a certain *dispositif* (apparatus) like psychiatry tries to align particular "truths" to its domain (Deleuze 1992; Foucault 2003). As such, psychiatric "truth" "is a truth which has its geography" (Foucault 2003, 236). The geography here is the MBU where a truth is "dispersed" across its space (Foucault 2003, 237). This is a "technology of demonstrative truth joined, in short, to scientific practice" (Foucault 2003, 236). This kind of "truth" uses the therapeutic process to produce a "cure" inside the "artificial locus" of the hospital walls (Foucault 1994, 17).

Despite the anti-psychiatry/critical psychiatry movement which emerged in the mid-twentieth century and contested psychiatry's strict alignment with scientific medical practices, claiming the need for a more human touch, women psychiatrists at Park House operate within particular regimes of truth (Breggin 1991; Cooper 2001; Foucault 1980; Laing 1967). This does not mean that conservative or traditional practices go uncontested, indeed the willingness of the all-women psychiatric team to participate in a study that interrogates the effectiveness of a purpose built MBU is testimony to their openness. Nonetheless, this may not be the case in other MBUs and "modern psychiatry [may still be] locked in a struggle with a rival will-to-truth which contest one another at every turn" (Kanyeredzi et al. 2019, 446). Even though it is the twenty-first century, institutional epistemologies and scientific "truths" operate with and against innovative approaches. The MBU is itself an innovative approach to the psychiatric care of mothers and babies and, as mentioned earlier, it has been established as best practice in many countries (Royal Australian & New Zealand College of Psychiatrists 2015). However, the built spaces need careful evaluation. Are they subscribing to old asylum-based "truths" or revised "truths"? We pick up these points further in chapter 3 where we show that the architects' intentions are to move as far away as possible from the prison and panoptic atmosphere of asylum design. For the architects to do this successfully, while ensuring the unit can provide the necessary therapeutic space, means that the architects need access to the "truths" of an MBU. Indeed, this is one of the main reasons for the research and the publication of this book.

Spatial, social, and clinical boundaries react with and against each other in an MBU. There are differing perceptions on the social contingencies of place, which Doreen Massey (1994, 136) elaborates on: "Localities, as I see them, are not just about the physical buildings, nor even about capital momentarily imprisoned; they are about the intersection of social activities and social relations and, crucially, activities and relations which are necessarily, by definition, dynamic, changing." Movement is never stable and movement in an MBU is linked to subjectivities, materialities, truths, and privacy. Mothers, toddlers, visitors, clinicians, student interns, cleaners, and researchers all move about, through, and within the MBU spaces in different ways at different times. These movements are not aimless such as may be found among people in an acute adult mental health unit, but purposeful. Even among very unwell mothers, task-related destinations are involved. However, in the design of the MBU used for this book, the way those destinations are reached provides some choices. As such, moving is a crucial part of a subject's conduct. However, despite the best of design intentions, interactions include the possibility of conflict even in generous spatial designs (Massey 1994). It is the ways that the spaces are settled in or moved through that is of particular interest. In a Foucauldian sense, it is through a study of the "conduct of conduct" that insights into movement in space are gained (Lemke 2015). This is because movements in a mental health unit can form a kind of "counter-conduct" (Foucault 2007, 191). As Foucault further writes (2007, 91), counter movements "are movements that also may seek, possibly at any rate, to escape direction by others and to define the way for each to conduct himself [*sic*]."

SUBJECT POSITIONING, TERMINOLOGY, AND LANGUAGE

How the subject might be formed and fractured, positioned and repositioned, is crucial to an understanding of all those involved in an MBU. We use the term subject in the Foucauldian sense of multiple subjects in one self. For example, there is the speaking subject, the productive subject, the economic subject, and the biological subject; each one can be objectified in particular scenarios (Foucault 1982). As such, there is the subject that is subjugated and subjected, but also the individual subject who struggles against forms of submission within her own self (Foucault 1982). Some questions on subjectivity that arise from this study include the following: How mothers position their subjectivity within a newly experienced liveable as opposed to an "unlivable" space (Butler 1993, 3); and how the simulated space of home reconstructs subjectivities of motherhood. In this way the MBU itself is a material intervention into subjectivities where life is precarious (Butler 2004).

In an MBU like the one that forms the case study for this book, there are not only the multiple subjects in a person who is unwell but also the multiple subjects in the staff and family, and the evolving subjectivities of the babies and toddlers (Rose 1999, 134). The roles of mother, nurse, psychologist, occupational therapist (and other therapists), psychiatrist, intern, medical student, mother-in-law, grandmother, grandfather, father, child, architect, and researcher are all problematized as they appear in the chapters. The main ones are addressed in some detail in the paragraphs that follow. To this extent subjectivities are rendered visible and inscribed in representational ways. A role-label is a social signifier and in some of those listed, also a professional signifier. Outer appearances are not necessarily an immediate signifier. Most nurses dressed in a similar type of casual uniform and it was difficult to tell the different types of nurses apart, which may have leveled otherwise visually obvious hierarchical staff divisions. Mothers, children, and their families were easier to identify, but psychiatrists, clinicians, and therapists who did not wear uniforms were at times also difficult to identify as they merged into the familial environment.

Writing about subjectification in a nonlinear way must necessarily recognize the "individualized, interiorized, totalized, and psychologized understanding of what it is to be human as the site of a historical problem" (Rose 1998, 18). Therefore, beneath, or perhaps above, visible signifiers is the affective human being; this resonates in the words of one mother in Park House: "When I first came here I didn't think I'd ever sort or warm to the staff, I really umm I really have. And I know that the staff, I'll miss the staff when I leave." The staff and other users of the MBU are overwhelmingly women compared to the architects who are men, which raises the question whether the shared gender of nurse and mother contributed to their bonding. The extent to which subjects in the MBU environment are gendered is of particular interest to us in this book.

Languages are integral to understanding how subjectivities are formed and subjectivities are at the heart of this book on mothers and their babies, away from home in institutional spaces. Therefore, what follows extends beyond a glossary and addresses the complicated relationship between language and ontology (Rose 1998). An MBU involves and includes a number of people, spaces, places, and activities; all are folded into each other in a Deleuzian sense (Rose 1998). Most of these are given different names across theory and practice, depending on context. The confusion which comes from differing terminology is significant, and goes well beyond being potentially confusing to also reflect the meanings inscribed. It references historical labeling and the dynamics of power relations in the mental health sector. Consequently, it is incumbent upon us as authors and researchers to explain our use of such terminology.

First, how might a person admitted to an MBU be referred to? There are several terms in use: historically it is "patient," often it is "client," and currently in Australian mental health services it is either "consumer" or "service user." In the forensic context, it has been "in-mate." In a documentary entitled *Mothers on the Edge* by Louis Theroux about mothers with postpartum psychosis in MBUs, Theroux uses "contributor" (Theroux 2019; for an analysis, see Riggs et al. 2020). None of these terms dignify the subjectivity of the human being. The mothers in the unit where our research for this book was conducted also referred to each other as "mothers" or more simply "mums," and the staff used the mothers' first names; but in discussion they were also referred to as "a mother." However, there were also fathers and grandmothers in the unit, and at times a father was admitted because he was also unwell. Additionally, a mother, being a mother, and mothering are not exclusively consigned to a female subject. Many children lose or are separated from their biological mothers, and mothering is taken up by another who may be of any gender (Chodorow 2012). In the professional sense one who is unwell and in a hospital in the care of the doctors and nurses may accept the term "patient." This could also be the case when visiting a general practitioner. Here the Lacanian subject expects to assume the understood role of "patient" in the language of medical practice. However, in an MBU, as in other mental health units, the subject may not accept that they are unwell. In this instance the label of patient is particularly disempowering. Conversely, if the subject in an MBU is called a "client," the language shifts ontologically to involve a set of different power relations. If the MBU is an exclusive private clinic, it may seem appropriate, but what of an MBU in the public health sector? A "client" may initiate the kind of assistance they are seeking, but they could also be referred to the MBU by a professional and/or not have had much choice. Either way, a service is implied and the interaction comes across as one where the expectation of what is required could be weighted toward the client and not the person offering the service. "Service user" could be even more depersonalizing than "client" both for the user and person providing the service; a transaction rather than a relationship is implied. And, if the service is provided online, human distancing is extreme. However, "service user" is the accepted term in mental health practice in Australia where our case study is based. "Consumer," the third in this trio of terms that mark the move away from "patient" sits even more firmly within a neoliberal language of economics.

Therefore, to return to the move away from "patient," perhaps something has been lost as well as gained in the attempt to empower the unwell person with a different type of label. Whatever the term, it is still a label and leaves us as authors in a quandary. We certainly do not use the demeaning term "in-mate," even though some of the mothers in a public health MBU are there by mental health order, but neither do we want to date our approach by only using the term "patient," and the other terms do not necessarily sit well with our own beliefs in empowering vulnerable subjectivities. Ultimately, we will be postmodern in our use of the language, and depending on the data we are drawing from, we will use "mother," "client," "service user," or "patient." While this may have the appearance of being inconsistent, it best represents the multiple ways that people in MBUs are positioned.

Second, different MBUs usually have an identifying name which can be after a philanthropist or another significant person. Mental health units broadly are typically disguised and given a name that does not have the stigma of "mental health" attached. This type of naming can be seen as lacking in transparency and contributing to the shame that some attach to being mentally unwell. Elsewhere we have written about a hospital mental health unit that decided to display the large identifying sign "Mental Health" specifically to emphasize the importance of this service in a suffering society. This suffering is a society with rising suicides and increasing poverty and homelessness all of which are related to mental health issues (Connellan, Due, and Riggs 2015; Ferguson et al. 2019). Clinical and administrative spaces are labeled in various ways that refer to their function either in a contemporary or historical way.

For the specific space in all mental health units and hospital wards which is called either the "Nurses' Station" or "Duty Station," we have selected "Nurses' Station" which is abbreviated to NS when it is used frequently in certain chapters. Despite the traditional and limiting aspects to the assignation, this space was consistently referred to as the Nurses' Station by everyone in the unit and is written as such in the field notes. More detail on the design, position, and naming of this somewhat contentious space is provided in chapter 3 "The Design: Architect Perspectives." This leads us also to the use of the term "nurse," which does not describe the very different roles of every mental health nurse who uses the space. It is not our intention to homogenize staff roles and when the field notes are clear, we refer to specific staff as psychiatrist, registrar, intern, or occupational therapist as shown. There are both gender and power problems with the term "nurse" which are not dissimilar to those discussed above with "mother." The generalization of "nurse" is of course not something we subscribe to but it is a term that was often innocently used by many participants in the study that forms the basis of this book. Many of the people in this book struggled with what was expected of them in their labeled roles within the environment of the MBU. Additionally, Park House is government funded which also brings a layer of bureaucracy, including adhering to assigned role-labels, which all staff are subject to, even if some of those rules are subjugating.

Finally, there are the subject positions of ourselves as authors of this book and researchers in the unit. There will be times when it is appropriate to use research language such as "interviewer" and "researcher" but if we were to use such academic language consistently, we would distance ourselves from the vulnerabilities of all participants who willingly shared with us and agreed to let us into their spaces.

There are four of us: Kathleen, Clemence, Damien, and Clare. Our collaboration stretches over a decade and has developed into a special relationship of trust and friendship. All of us are the child of a mother, and have experienced mothering in different ways and places. Some of us have our own children, and collectively we watch them all grow, each in their wonderfully unique way. As lead author, the others have sometimes referred to the book as "my baby," but together we share the pain and joy of its labor. Our individual biographies will tell you a little more about each of us.

As observational ethnographers in an MBU, we were aware that even when the mother-child relationship is tested beyond the boundaries of the known, there is always hope. Sitting in the spaces that sometimes streamed with natural light and seemed to beam encouragement on the mothers and their babies, we watched, waited, looked on, and took notes with care. If our presence began to weigh heavily in the space, we quietly moved away to give the mothers their privacy. In the interview situation, we asked and listened, trying to ensure that the mother, partner, grandmother, or clinician could share what they thought and felt about the spaces designed for them. To be in the position of asking questions and recording the responses is to be in a position of privilege, but also one of enormous responsibility. We were trusted to be with vulnerable women and with passionately dedicated clinicians; they wanted to tell their story so that the public may know the immense importance of good design.

CHAPTER SUMMARIES

In this chapter we provided a detailed introduction that sets the book's conceptual framework of gender, space, and health. It plunges into the space of a contemporary MBU with an opening anecdote from a mother, reminding the reader that this book is about mothers who are psychologically fragile and require a suitably designed space to heal and nurture their mother-child relationship. This is followed by casting back briefly to the departure from asylums and mother-baby separation with the rise of MBUs. The chapter also clarifies that the book is concerned with the effect upon all users of the MBU space, which crucially includes staff and families. Four research questions are laid out in this chapter: (1) How can built space affect the relationships and interaction between staff and clients? (2) How can built space affect the work and well-being of staff? (3) How can built space affect interactions between clients and their families? and (4) How can built space impact on clients, staff, and families in terms of gender and other aspects of identity (e.g., culture or age)? The chapter explains that the case study of a contemporary MBU provides the empirical framework for the book. Chapter 1 positions the book within a broadly based feminist discourse. As such, this chapter questions normative understandings of a "mother" and discusses misconceptions regarding binary divisions of male and female both psychologically and architecturally. Following this gender foregrounding, fundamental concepts of privacy and regulation culminate with an open discussion on subject positioning, terminology, and language. The chapter draws upon the work of authors such as Kate Boyer, Doreen Massey, Michel Foucault, and Nicholas Rose, as well as our own previous publications.

Chapter 2 provides a context for the book, providing an overview of MBUs and existing research, alongside details of the case study upon which the book is based. The first half of the chapter provides a historical background to the emergence of MBUs, then provides a review of the research into MBUs across the past few decades. Key and secondary themes from the research into MBUs are foregrounded in the review section, focusing on admissions data from MBUs; outcomes for mothers and babies; programs and interventions; follow up after discharge; separation of mothers and babies after discharge; client satisfaction with MBUs; and partners of women admitted to MBUs. The majority of the studies included in this review section are quantitative and the need for more qualitative work is recommended to provide more context and connections, especially in relation to design and setting. The second half of the chapter is devoted to an explanation of our case study which is specifically about architectural design for facilities for mothers and babies in need of psychiatric support and intervention. The setting and facilities of the MBU in the case study are described in detail. This is followed by a detailed description of the ethnographic observations and interviews undertaken.

Chapter 3 centers upon the architects' perspectives in the design of the MBU. As such, the data drawn upon for the chapter are taken chiefly from architect interview transcripts and design briefs and plans. However, to support the argument that detailed practical use of the spaces requires consistent architect consideration, some interview data from clients as well as ethnographic observational data are also used. The chapter considers the role of male architects leading the design of an MBU for users who are overwhelmingly female. The chapter is structured according to themes arising from the architects' data and include the following: evidence-based design; consultation processes; successes and challenges of the designs; the old mortuary; model of care; movement; gardens; safety/privacy; and domesticity. Of these themes, the problems which arose from protracted, but underrepresented, consultation in the design briefing emerged as the strongest factor. The central private gardens are evaluated for their success in the design, as is the effect of movement in the positioning of the open-plan/thoroughfare dining area. The old model of care which required clear lines of sight is shown to be partially subverted by the design, but the chapter considers how this works in the reality of the space. The central idea of homelike versus institutional design is shown to be ambivalent. The chapter is longer than other chapters given that it is specifically about the design and the architectural angle, which is the book's focus. The chapter is also illustrated with several images from the unit which emphasize the design's influence on practicalities among staff and clients.

Chapter 4 enters into the built space of the MBU which we have called "Park House." Drawing specifically upon the ethnographic observational data, the functioning and use of the space is examined with a keen focus on the effects that the space appeared to produce. This chapter allows the reader to inhabit the space with the ethnographers so that liminal aspects such as light, sound, conviviality, and homeliness are understood. These ambient aspects are situated within the more structural spatial parameters. The chapter is a reflexive critique, therefore the difficulty and perhaps impossibility of neutral observation runs through all the themes. These themes are consequently analyzed in a specifically situated manner with the ambivalences of insider and outsider providing a necessary friction. As such, practices of observation and surveillance are scrutinized from the design and placement of: glazing, monitors, doors, and sleep, play and eating areas. The chapter provides illustrative detail of materialities so that clicking shoes, crying babies, and mixing milk formula is heard and sensed in the interrogation of functioning spaces. There are spaces that are used for routine activities, alongside other spaces that may invite mothers to linger. This chapter is as much about the design as it is about the intense human needs within it. The subheadings of: Light and Sound; Practices of observation and surveillance; The Use of the Space; Mealtimes; Conviviality; Effects of the Space; Homeliness; conclude with the theme of our book which is "home and away from home." How the determined veneer of homeliness operates alongside clinical care and abiding observation is a constant reminder of Park House as "away."

Chapter 5 draws upon the data from staff interviews with a focus on how they perceived and experienced the design of the MBU, and how it worked for both them and those in their care. Substantial excerpts from the data are quoted and thematically analyzed. The chapter identifies the following eight overarching themes and deals with them sequentially—Staff Experiences; Privacy versus Clinical Needs; The Therapeutic Space: Accommodating Therapy; Creating Home in an Institution; Smoking; Noise; Accommodating Children in an MBU; and Flexible Outdoor Spaces Facilitate Parent-Child Relationships. All staff interviews were with women and their interview data are chiefly about the mothers and their mental health needs. The first theme shows staff commenting on shortcomings regarding space and confidentiality in the nurses' station, puzzlement at the light orientation, but overall satisfaction with the size and design of the unit. The second theme includes crucial comments regarding bedrooms, psychological space, and individual needs. With regard to the theme on therapeutic space requirements, the walk-throughs and opportunities for apparently casual, but nonetheless important, exchanges with mothers are abundantly clear. However, this satisfaction sits ambivalently with the need to go through locked doors to reach some interview rooms, where the relaxed approach is undermined. Being at home in an institution was an important element of staff perspective, with the "attractive" design implied as a means of reducing stigma. The chapter shows staff speaking to the delicate aspect of being too at home and not wanting to leave while at the same time needing to prepare service users for exactly that. Other challenges come up in the themes of smoking and noise. Many mothers needed to smoke and this created security issues, particularly at night, as smoking was not allowed on hospital grounds; the chapter speaks to the difficulties raised by staff who were both sensitive to this "legal" drug, aware of its addictive qualities, and cognizant of why anxious mothers were dependent upon it. Noise and sound is also raised by staff who note the shortage of nurseries, the noise of alarms, the location of the laundry opposite to the nurseries, and the impossibility of picking up monitor sounds if staff are not in the nurses' station. Quoted excerpts are explicit about potential safety issues if calls are not heard. The last theme on accommodating children shows that the unit does not serve all ages (zero months to three years) adequately with insufficient nurseries, insufficient play space for toddlers, and some design elements which did not meet the needs of mothers learning to raise their children. Despite some reservations around heat in summer, the chapter reveals most staff thought the garden areas afforded many opportunities for relationship building. Overall, the chapter presents an important perspective on the space within the unit—particularly regarding the unique needs of mothers and their children within such units, which may not be well understood by those who do not intimately understand these needs leading to subsequent issues in design.

Chapter 6 uses the data from interviews with the clients/service users who are predominantly mothers, with one grandmother and two partners. These interviews took place in ways which did not interrupt what the mothers were doing at the time; as such, some interviews took place in the dining area, with children present, in groups of other people, and with their partner. As such, while the verbal components of these interviews are important and form the basis of the analysis in this chapter, the interviews also occurred in ways that helped to demonstrate the service users' experience of the spaces. Chapter 6 brings this informal approach alive with substantive excerpts accompanied by analysis, all of which are grouped into four themes: Homeliness; Tensions concerning Privacy: Isolation, Security, and Assistance; Spaces Facilitating Relationships; and Spaces for Sleep as Less than Ideal. Welcoming and friendly aspects that contributed to homeliness were discussed by the service users alongside interruptions to homeliness, such as controlled air conditioning. Distinctions between hospital-like atmosphere and homely atmosphere are expressed with clarity, however there are differences of opinion: what seems quiet and private to some is not perceived as such by others. A key issue is the need to be safe but not isolated. Most clients/service users welcome the light-filled spaces and the opportunities for developing relationships with their children in the gardens and shared spaces, but others do not feel comfortable doing this in view of others, leading to some mothers potentially becoming isolated as they remain in their bedrooms as much as possible. Service users pointed out the spatial challenges for children of different ages, which made some areas unsafe for little babies and toddlers together. The chapter highlights the spatial divide between the private bedroom and communal or shared spaces, for example there is no choice but to leave the bedroom to prepare baby formula. As such, the design dictates a departure from what could be a depressed psychological space in the interior of a room to the demands of functioning in an exterior shared by staff and other mothers. The chapter shows that all service users were impressed with the unobtrusive assistance provided by staff, with excerpts and analysis indicating that the open-plan light-filled spaces facilitated this. Nonetheless, adequate sleep—that all important requirement for the mothers and babies' progress—is a key aspect where design provision falls short. Noise and light are identified as interrupting sleep, especially with insufficient nursery space. The service users' opinions and experiences of a space that is specifically designed for them to become well together with their babies is a crucial part of this book and this chapter shows how intricately spatial materialities coalesce or jar with their development.

Chapter 7 does more than summarize the book, it extends the book's interrogation of space to explore how people and space intersect in Park House and MBUs more broadly. The chapter posits that designed space offers cues for human behavior and it takes up several of these cues. The space provided opportunities for us as ethnographers and researchers to read the cues and this final chapter identifies them as firstly "dys/regulated spaces" situated in the following ways: fraught, sensory, and developmentalist. The spaces are fraught with competing requirements between "home" and institution; they are sensory-filled spaces resonant with smells, noises, and light changes, all potentially triggering sensory reactions or overload; they are spaces for developing mother-child relationships and healthy attachment. Second, the spaces are situated as "peopled spaces" providing cues for normative gendering and challenges for cultural and other forms of diversity, including the prohibition of nonhuman animal family members known to facilitate good mental health outcomes. Third, the spaces are cued as "imagined" in a way that is at once homely but also temporary, therefore providing tensions between the comfort of being safe but knowing that it is conditional and transient. Lastly, the spaces are firmly and visibly situated as "healthy spaces" which resonates with institutional legibility but the chapter problematizes notions of design for health from the view of building relationships and points to those areas that require more research. All these cues are provided and made legible through the subjectivities of us as researchers and others as staff and service users, but the chapter emphasizes that the cues do not provide a predetermined reading.

Chapter 2

An Overview of Psychiatric Mother-Baby Unit Research

Since as early as the 1970s theorists have pointed toward the need to move away from a model of health care premised upon managing disease, and toward one that focuses on the factors that maintain and promote good health. One of the key changes in mental health design has been the move from asylums to the design of mental health care facilities that attempt to simulate a domestic environment. This shift aims to serve those who occupy them (including clients and staff) by providing a less obviously institutional space. In terms of psychiatric care for mothers, this led to a move away from the practice of separating mothers and babies when mothers require psychiatric treatment, to the creation of purpose built MBUs. Despite there now existing a large body of work theorizing the forms that such new approaches to mental health design might take, there has been little empirical research undertaken on how purpose built design in mental health works in practice. More specifically, there are a growing number of studies examining MBUs, but these rarely consider the impact of the built space on staff, client, and visitor experiences, and how space impacts on mental health outcomes.

This chapter consists of two parts. The first part provides a brief background to MBUs before providing a review of existing research about MBUs, with a focus on key themes and findings. The second part of the chapter details the MBU case study drawn on throughout the book, providing a background to the setting and methods used in the study.

BACKGROUND TO PSYCHIATRIC MOTHER-BABY UNITS

As a background, it is important to note the high rates of significant mental health conditions experienced by women in the postpartum period and hence the need for psychiatric care, including MBUs. For women who give birth to children the early postpartum period presents the greatest risk of severe psychiatric disorder and admission to psychiatric services for this population than any other period of their lives (Cantwell 2016). Reviews indicate that 15–20 percent of all women in the perinatal period are affected by a significant mental health condition (Sutter-Dallay and Guedeney 2016). Suicide attempts can also be high during the postpartum period (Gressier et al. 2017). Importantly, women can be affected by preexisting mental health conditions (e.g., schizophrenia, bipolar affective disorder, depressive and anxiety disorders, eating disorders, substance misuse disorders, and personality disorders) and/or mental health conditions arising in the postpartum period (e.g., postpartum psychosis and postnatal depression) (Cantwell 2016).

During the first half of the twentieth century, the separation of mothers and their babies was viewed as best practice when mothers were experiencing severe forms of mental illness and required psychiatric treatment. Howard (2000) notes that mothers viewed as requiring treatment tended to be admitted without their babies to institutions or asylums, particularly at the height of their usage in the early decades of the twentieth century. The practice of separating mothers and babies began to change, however, during the 1950s and 1960s, when research findings indicated that keeping mothers and babies together was best for establishing a secure mother-child relationship (Howard 2000) and this began to appear in practice (e.g., Douglas 1956; Main 1958). This led to the creation of psychiatric inpatient mother-baby units, which appeared in some form in the late 1950s and early 1960s in the UK (Baker et al. 1961). The first MBU in France opened in 1979 in Créteil followed by three more in the 1980s (Cazas and Glangeaud-Freudenthal 2004), though joint mother-baby inpatient admissions occurred in France as early as 1960 (Baker et al. 1961). The 1980s saw the establishment of MBUs in Australia (in Melbourne in 1983) (Buist et al. 2004) and in Belgium (in Zoersel in 1985) (Glangeaud-Freudenthal et al. 2014). Since then, MBUs have opened in a number of other countries around the world.

MBUs appeared in the context of a range of social changes and research advances, including new understandings concerning the importance of the mother-baby relationship and attachment (e.g., Bowlby 1969), advances in relevant psychiatric treatments, the changing nature of asylums (directed by government policy), changing family structures (meaning that other carers were often not available), the development of social psychiatry, and the increase in the number of psychiatrists who were women (Cazas and Glangeaud-Freudenthal 2004; Howard 2000). MBUs are now viewed as the best setting for mothers with severe mental illness in several countries, given co-admission potentially reduces interruptions to attachment relationships (e.g., Cazas and Glangeaud-Freudenthal 2004; Green et al. 2016; National Institute for Health and Care Excellence 2014; Royal Australian & New Zealand College of Psychiatrists 2015).

The countries that have most actively promoted MBUs include the UK, Australia, France, and Belgium, which is reflected by the higher number of MBUs in those locations. MBUs have also been established in other European countries including Belgium (e.g., Glangeaud-Freudenthal and The MBU-SMF Working Group 2004), the Netherlands (Noorlander et al. 2008), Hungary (Glangeaud-Freudenthal et al. 2014), and Germany (Grube 2005), and outside Europe in the United States (Meltzer-Brody et al. 2014), Israel (Maizel et al. 2005), India (Chandra et al. 2015), Sri Lanka (Glangeaud-Freudenthal et al. 2014), and New Zealand (Cazas and Glangeaud-Freudenthal 2004). Practices and admissions differ between (and within) countries, however, due to different mental health and perinatal care systems within each location and the fact that they may cater for clients presenting with different mental health issues (Glangeaud-Freudenthal and The MBU-SMF Working Group 2004). The existence of individual MBUs can be tenuous, and numbers have fluctuated due to a range of factors including funding, the interest of doctors (who are largely responsible for keeping the units in existence), whether children are considered patients or not, and the size of the unit (Cazas and Glangeaud-Freudenthal 2004). While MBUs are financially costly to run, the outcomes achieved in this service reduce the likelihood of future issues and replace the need for future costs in relation to other psychiatric services for mothers, child welfare services, and issues relating to the impact of child mental health on child development (Bauer et al. 2014; Glangeaud-Freudenthal et al. 2016).

While MBUs are now established best practice in many countries, there is no accepted definition of how an MBU should be structured or run (Elkin et al. 2009). Generally, psychiatric inpatient MBUs refer to separate wards or buildings dedicated to housing mothers and their babies full-time, with at least four beds and cots or bassinettes (Elkin et al. 2009; Glangeaud-Freudenthal et al. 2014). MBUs are usually staffed by multidisciplinary teams whose role is to care for mothers and babies, with expertise focused on the treatment of mothers' mental health conditions, building attachment relationships and positive interactions between mothers and babies, and assisting mothers to gain skills in child care and development (Glangeaud-Freudenthal et al. 2014).

Review of Existing Research on Psychiatric Mother-Baby Units

In this section we draw on a review we undertook of the literature on MBUs to provide an overall picture of recent empirical research which has been conducted in and about MBUs around the world (for our earlier systematic review, see Connellan, Bartholomaeus, Due, and Riggs 2017). Three key themes predominated across the studies (1) admissions data, (2) outcomes for mothers and babies, and (3) the impact of programs and interventions in MBUs. Four secondary themes were represented in the studies: (i) follow-up after discharge, (ii) separation of mothers and babies after discharge, (iii) client satisfaction of MBU, and (iv) partners of women admitted to MBUs. Additional sources focused on understanding the characteristics of the populations admitted to MBUs. In terms of location, most studies focused on MBUs in the UK and Australia. This concentration on the UK and Australia can be understood both by the prominence of MBUs in these locations and our focus on English-language publications. Research also related to MBUs located in Belgium, France, Germany, India, Israel, the Netherlands, and the United States.

Key Theme 1: Admissions Data from MBUs

Several sources provide detailed information about admissions to MBUs, including number of joint admissions, maternal age, infant age, primary diagnosis, length of stay, and, in some cases, ethnic and/or socioeconomic backgrounds of mothers. Maternal mean age ranged from 24.25 years (Chandra et al. 2015) to 33.5 years (Christl et al. 2015), and infant mean age at time of admission ranged from 9.6 weeks (Glangeaud-Freudenthal et al. 2011, 2013) to 7.82 months (Yelland et al. 2015). Mean length of stay ranged from 6.93 days in a study from the United States (Meltzer-Brody et al. 2014) to 11.6 weeks in a study in Israel (Maizel et al. 2005). These differences are likely to be, at least in part, due to the different nature and purpose of MBUs in different locations.

Primary diagnosis for mothers varied greatly between the MBUs, again, likely a reflection of the varying nature and purpose of MBUs. The most common diagnoses overall were depressive illnesses, schizophrenia, and differing forms of psychosis.

Key Theme 2: Outcomes for Mothers and Babies

Overall, studies focused on outcomes for mothers suggest that the mental health of mothers who are admitted to MBUs improves significantly by the time they are discharged. The largest study conducted on outcomes was undertaken by Salmon et al. (2003), who analyzed the outcomes of 1,081 women in eight MBUs in the UK and found that 78 percent were symptom-free or considerably improved in terms of maternal clinical outcome, and most scored at least 80 percent on three parenting outcomes. Women with schizophrenia, however, had poorer outcomes on all measures. Abel et al. (2005), who used admissions data to relate predictors to outcomes, found that protective factors such as social stability among women with schizophrenia enhance successful parenting in this group. Gillham and Wittkowski (2015) have written a systematic review of outcomes for women admitted to MBUs. One of their key findings was the women with a diagnosis of schizophrenia had less positive outcomes from MBU admissions.

Glangeaud-Freudenthal et al. (2011) in their analysis of 869 women in 13 MBUs in France found that two-thirds (69 percent) of the women were symptom-free or considerably improved by the time they were discharged, with this being higher for those with issues appearing (or reappearing) in the postpartum period compared to those with chronic mental illness. Other studies have also shown improved outcomes for mothers and babies as a result of MBUs (Hill et al. 2019; Le Treut et al. 2018; Stephenson et al. 2018), although in some cases babies have been found to have developmental and mental health concerns (Wright, Stevens, and Wouldes 2018).

Key Theme 3: Programs and Interventions in MBUs

Some of the sources have a strong focus on interventions that enable parenting skills and emotionally responsive mother-infant interactions. In terms of specific findings, Butler et al. (2014) examined the views of mothers about a parenting program (the Baby Triple P Positive Parenting Program) run in one UK MBU. The mothers viewed the program as beneficial, and the MBU as a good setting to engage in the program, although it was noted that a commitment to the program may be difficult for mothers recovering from mental health issues. Additionally, some of those mothers said that MBU staff needed to be more familiar with the program. Butler (2013) also examined the views of staff in an MBU about the same parenting program, finding that they too viewed the program as a positive intervention and the MBU as a useful setting for it (see also Butler-Coyne et al. 2017).

Bilszta et al. (2012) examined the potential usefulness of video-only feedback or verbal-only feedback interventions in comparison with standard care to improve maternal parenting among women in an Australian MBU. They found that the interventions were not clearly better than standard care (which already include music and art therapy interventions). A video feedback intervention was also used by Kenny et al. (2013) in the UK to examine possibilities for improving mother-infant interaction. They found that there were improved interactions regardless of the diagnoses (including schizophrenia) of the mothers. In Belgium, Van Puyvelde et al. (2014) examined the potential for mother-infant group therapy using music to establish maternal-infant intersubjectivity. They found that maternal-infant intersubjectivity increased from Session 1 to Session 5, although their findings are based on a small sample. Similarly, Reilly et al. (2019) piloted a singing intervention in Australia. They found positive changes in self-reported mood state when comparing pre- and post-session.

Other studies have considered interventions in MBUs more broadly. For example, Garrett, Turner, and Wittkowski (2018) surveyed ten MBUs in the UK and found that most offered multiple psychological interventions as well as individual therapy. In addition, Korteland et al. (2019) examined nursing interventions for women with postpartum psychosis in an MBU in the Netherlands, finding that nurses described tailoring these interventions to the needs of particular patients, babies, and partners.

Secondary Theme I: Follow-up after Discharge from MBU

A small number of sources explicitly focused on follow-up and outcomes following discharge from an MBU. A three-and-a-half-year follow-up study in Belgium found that 61 percent of mothers were functioning "relatively well," but 39 percent continued to be impacted by severe depression (Vliegen et al. 2010, 2013). In the UK, Hipwell et al.'s (2000) follow-up study of eighty-two mother-infant dyads over the child's first year of life found that mother-infant interactions were still impacted negatively by the mother's illness. Also, in the UK, a follow-up study of children aged four to six whose mothers had previously been MBU inpatients and who were currently living with that mother, were not found to have poorer developmental outcomes with comparison children or standardized child norms, although some had issues with attachment (Wan et al. 2007).

One of the few qualitative studies about MBUs examines eight women's lived experiences following discharge from an MBU in Australia (Connerty et al. 2016). This study is important as it provides information to assist in understanding outcomes reported in quantitative studies. The study found that the women experienced returning home from the MBU as a significant life event and that women did not feel they had clear support plans post-discharge. Howard et al. (2003) use data from 1,255 mothers on the Marcé database in 2001 to ascertain levels of continued social service supervision after discharge, noting that mothers with schizophrenia show a high risk of supervision and recommending that the whole family context should be treated.

Secondary Theme II: Separation of Mothers and Children at Discharge from MBU

There are also a small number of sources which examine the separation of mothers and children at discharge from an MBU. Two large studies of over 1,000 mother/child pairings have been conducted (Glangeaud-Freudenthal et al. 2013; Howard et al. 2003), as well as a number of smaller studies. Glangeaud-Freudenthal et al.'s (2013) prospective longitudinal study of 1,018 women in France and Belgium found that most children were discharged with their mothers, but that 151 (14.8 percent) were separated at discharge. Of those separated, 41 percent of children were placed in foster families, 41 percent in institutions, 13 percent with family members (3 percent with fathers), and 1 percent stayed at the MBU for more than a month after the mother was discharged. Glangeaud-Freudenthal et al. (2013) argue that there were a number of risk factors for separation: babies with medical complications, type of psychiatric disorder for mothers, type of psychiatric disorder for fathers, mothers' lack of good social relationships with others, mothers receiving disability benefits, and low socioeconomic class. Additionally, Glangeaud-Freudenthal et al.'s study highlights the connection between the child's vulnerability and the existence of the above-listed factors, such as maternal and paternal mental health and psychosocial contexts. Drawing specifically on data from 320 women suffering from a psychotic disorder and jointly admitted to an MBU in France or Belgium between 2001 and 2010, Cès et al. (2018) found that a higher number of mothers and infants were separated at discharge (27.2 percent).

Howard et al.'s (2003) analysis of the data of mothers entered on the Marcé database in the UK identified data relating to discharge for 1,197 women. In terms of discharges, 77 percent (921) of babies were discharged with their mother without formal supervision. Of the 23 percent discharged with their babies under a form of social services supervision or without their babies, 6 percent (75) of all babies were discharged with mothers placed on an "at risk" register, 7 percent (81) were discharged with mothers under a protection or care order, 6 percent (69) were placed in voluntary foster care, and 4 percent (51) were placed in statutory care or adopted. There was an increased risk of social services supervision for mothers with schizophrenia and personality disorder, as well as in relation to social class, single marital status, behavioral disturbance, and psychiatric illness in partners. Smaller studies have also found that the type of mental health diagnosis is a key factor in separation at discharge (e.g., Poinso et al. 2002; Seneviratne, Conroy, and Marks 2003).

Secondary Theme III: Client Satisfaction with MBUs

The few studies examining client satisfaction with MBUs found experiences to be generally positive overall, including the finding that MBUs are preferable to general psychiatric wards. However, existing studies have small sample sizes. Neil, Sanderson, and Wieck (2006) developed the Mother and Baby Unit Satisfaction Questionnaire, but note that it is limited because service users were not formally consulted in its development. Their study in the UK of twenty women found overall satisfaction to be high and that the MBU was preferred over a general psychiatric ward. Women were most satisfied with baby equipment (very satisfied 85 percent), visitor arrangements for partners/relatives (63.2 percent), partner involvement with baby (63.2 percent), appearance of the ward (65.0 percent), privacy (60 percent), and waiting times (57.9 percent). Women were least satisfied with involvement in their own care (very or quite dissatisfied 50 percent) and organized activities (47.4 percent).

A modified version of the Mother and Baby Unit Satisfaction Questionnaire was used by Antonysamy et al. (2009), also in the UK. Their survey of fifty-seven women found that 84.2 percent were satisfied overall with the MBU. Over 90 percent were satisfied with baby care advice (96.4 percent), baby equipment (94.8 percent), and advice on child development (94.7 percent). Mothers were most dissatisfied with organized activities (33.4 percent) and food (17.6 percent). Interviews in the same study found that all women preferred the MBU to general psychiatric wards because they viewed it as more secure and thought it was important to be with their baby to help with recovery. Some mothers also said that they had insufficient access to doctors and nursing staff.

Similar findings are evident from Nair et al. (2010) telephone survey of thirty-seven women in Australia who had previously been admitted to an MBU. Sixty percent of women said admission to the MBU was "very" or "quite" useful, but noted that areas to improve included increased staff availability (27 percent), staff behavior (22 percent), and increased practical support availability (19 percent).

Crocker (2013–2014) piloted the Patient Rated Outcome and Experience Measure (PROM) in MBUs in the UK. Of the sixty-eight respondents who completed the measure across six MBUs, over 90 percent were satisfied with thirteen of the seventeen questions relating to satisfaction. Low levels of satisfaction related to organization of discharge (7.4 percent dissatisfied) and how quickly help was received after referral (7.4 percent).

A qualitative study in a newly developed MBU in New Zealand (Wright, Jowsey et al. 2018) found that mothers were positive about several aspects, including being admitted with their infants, interactions with staff, and involvement of partners and family. Another study in the UK explored the importance of compassionate care for women admitted to MBUs (Wittkowski, Hare, and Gillham 2019).

Secondary Theme IV: Male Partners of Women Admitted to MBUs

There are also only a small number of studies focused on partners of women admitted to MBUs (all focused on male partners), although this topic is also mentioned in some additional sources. Of the studies where partners were a primary focus, Grube's (2005) German study with thirty-one male partners of women admitted to MBUs found that only a third of partners could be described as "supportive" (a "competent father," "supportive partner," and "having a symmetric relationship") and that women with supportive male partners had a shorter stay in the MBU. Grube's study also highlights the high rate of male partners with psychiatric disorders.

Kemp's (2011) qualitative interview study with six fathers in the UK found that fathers tried to make sense of what had happened to their partner, felt limited in being able to help, faced competing physical and emotional demands of partner, child and self, had their role and identity challenged by the MBU, and viewed that treatment should be family-focused (including fathers). Similarly, Boddy et al. (2017) explored the experiences of seven fathers whose partners had been admitted to two MBUs in the UK. Their findings focus on men's confusion and difficulty in relation to their partners' postpartum psychosis and admission to MBUs. Other UK research also focuses on the difficulties men encounter when their partner has been admitted to an MBU (Marrs et al. 2014; Reid et al. 2017).

Finally, Turner, Garrett, and Wittkowski (2018) surveyed ten MBUs in the UK to explore the support they offered to partners of women admitted to MBUs. They found that while all of the MBUs who completed the survey offered support to male partners, additional support was suggested in the forms of peer support groups, information/skills groups targeted at partners, and therapy for individuals and couples.

AN OVERVIEW OF THE PSYCHIATRIC MOTHER-BABY UNIT CASE STUDY

This book draws on a case study of an MBU in Australia. As mentioned above, Australia is one of the countries where MBUs are most promoted. MBUs have been advocated for in the Recommendations from The Royal Australian & New Zealand College of Psychiatrists (RANZCP) since 2007, although they note that this is "not always feasible":

> The RANZCP supports admission to mother-and-baby psychiatric units with appropriately trained staff as best practice. General adult psychiatric facilities are not an appropriate environment for infants and do not have the requisite parenting facilities or specialist expertise. The RANZCP acknowledges however

> that admission to mother-and-baby psychiatric units is not always feasible in every jurisdiction across Australia and New Zealand currently. (2015, 2)

The first MBU as such opened in Australia in 1983 at Larundel Psychiatric Hospital in Melbourne, Victoria as a two-bed unit (Buist, Dennerstein, and Burrows 1990; Buist et al. 2004). Since then, MBUs have opened in all major cities across Australia, although many are private and therefore are not accessible to all mothers and their babies (Brockington, Butterworth, and Glangeaud-Freudenthal 2017, 114). A recent review of five public MBUs in Australia showed that they follow very similar admission criteria, although differ slightly in aspects including number of admissions, mean length of stay, and the professions of staff (e.g., number of psychiatric nursing staff) (Galbally et al. 2019).

Setting

The present study was conducted in a government-run MBU in Australia. The purpose built unit opened in December 2012, and replaced a previous facility, originally opened in 1981 as a Family Unit. The purpose of the unit is to provide inpatient psychiatric services for mothers who experience mental health concerns postpartum (including puerperal psychosis, bipolar mood disorder, schizophrenia, schizo-affective disorder, major depressive disorder, or severe anxiety disorders; additionally, dual diagnoses may include a primary mental health problem or current substance misuse). As such, the mother is the client of the unit, though given the practice of co-admission, the child/ren and potentially partner may also receive treatment. Partners may also stay overnight in the unit, which is unusual compared to most MBUs around the world (Glangeaud-Freudenthal et al. 2016). The unit also provides outpatient services to mothers who have previously been admitted to the unit. Mothers are usually admitted with one or more of their babies/children under three years old (which differs from many other MBUs in Australia which limit child admissions to under twelve months old). Mothers are referred to the inpatient unit by a medical practitioner or a mental health clinician and in some cases mothers are admitted on a mental health order. The unit is publicly funded and staying at the unit is free of charge for mothers and their babies. The average length of time that each mother and baby stays at the unit is three weeks, although this varies depending on the support and treatment required. While the MBU is technically for parents (rather than only mothers) and their babies, during our period of observations no fathers were admitted as clients (although we were told by unit staff that in the past a father who was a primary caregiver had been admitted, and that more recently both a mother and a father had been admitted together, along with their child).

In terms of design, the MBU has four family and two single bedrooms, all with en suite bathrooms. The MBU also has three shared nurseries to accommodate sleeping babies. Clients have available to them a range of shared spaces including a large dining area and a beverage and snack preparation area, a kitchen, an infant formula room, two lounge rooms, a laundry, and an enclosed play area with toys for children. The entire unit is built around two gardens with play equipment, seating, and space for barbeques. More details on the design are provided in chapter 3.

With regard to the operations of the MBU, mothers are expected to be the main carer for their child/ren, depending on their mental and physical health, with staff providing support 24/7 and helping mothers develop the skills needed in order to leave the unit. Mothers are expected to be responsible for feeding their baby, cleaning up after their baby, and doing their own laundry, again depending on their mental and physical health. Mothers are allowed visits from family (including children over three years old) and friends. The unit provides breakfast, lunch, and dinner each day for mothers, linen, and baby equipment (e.g., cots, high chairs, prams). Mothers are required to bring clothes for themselves and their baby, and toiletries, nappies, and formula/food if required.

In terms of staffing, the unit has a multidisciplinary team comprised of nurses (day and night) including mental health nurses, psychiatrists, a psychiatry registrar, a pediatric registrar, a clinical psychologist, a mother-infant therapist (who works specifically on facilitating attachment), a social worker, and other support staff, including Patient Services Assistants, occupational therapists, and music and art therapists. The unit often includes university students on placement (e.g., medical and nursing students) and a number of cleaners who are employed by the broader hospital network of which the unit is a part. As part of the integrated model of care adopted within the unit, mothers and babies are provided with medical and therapeutic support during their stay and a discharge plan for when they leave. Apart from medication management and access to electroconvulsive therapy offsite (if required), key specialist service interventions address the mental health, psychosocial and emotional needs of the mother-infant relationship. Group programs use a range of therapeutic modalities including partner and family counseling, cognitive behavior therapy (CBT), music, art, journaling, psycho-educational groups, practical parenting and skills development, and diversional fitness groups. Many of these programs include partners (where relevant) to re-establish parent-child attachment. Care plans typically involve the family at all stages of treatment, beginning with the initial assessment, which is then tailored for individuals and supported by social workers up to and crucially including the discharge plan.

Methods

We conducted a comprehensive case study of the MBU, bringing together ethnographic observations of the MBU, and interviews with architects, staff, and clients and partners/family members. As far as we are aware, only one previous study of an MBU has involved an ethnography (Masciantonio 2015), and no studies have interviewed architects about their involvement in MBU design. Previous research with staff, clients, and partners in relation to MBUs has not specifically explored the built space and design, and is often quantitative in design.

Ethics approval for the research was granted from the first author's University ethics committee and the research ethics committee of the broader hospital network. Prior to the start of the ethnographic observations, the first and fourth authors presented information about the research to a large group of the MBU staff. Information sheets about the study were also displayed in the nurses' station. Clients were told about the research by staff and were given an information sheet and consent form to sign if they agreed to be included in the ethnographic observations. During the observational period of the research two mothers did not wish to be observed, so no notes were taken about them. Due to ethics constraints, it was not possible to ask the mothers why they declined to participate. All interview participants were given information sheets and consent forms to sign.

Ethnographic Observations

The ethnographic observations focused on how people in the unit moved in and interacted with the space. Ethnography has been used previously in mental health settings (Johansson, Skärsäter, and Danielson 2006; Savage 2000; Sinding 2010), including in our own research (Due, Connellan and Riggs 2012; Riggs, Due, and Connellan 2013; Connellan, Due, and Riggs 2015), and was thus considered to be an appropriate methodology for use in this study.

A total of thirty hours of ethnographic observations were conducted by the first and fourth authors in May-June 2015. The fourth author carried out ethnographic observations on eleven separate days for two hours each visit (total twenty-two hours). These observations occurred at various times between 8.30 a.m. and 6:00 p.m. on weekdays. Following this, the first author visited an additional four times for two hours each visit, in the afternoon, evening, and night on three weekdays (at various times from 4:00 p.m. to midnight) and a late Sunday afternoon. These relatively short two-hour blocks of observations were used both to reduce the "burden" on the MBU and its users and to ensure we remained as focused as possible in our observations. Observations were conducted in various locations in client, staff, and shared spaces, particularly in the dining area and the nurses' station. Additional observations were conducted in spaces including the main client lounge, the acute client lounge, the corridor near the nurseries, the central garden, and the corridor in the staff-only section. For privacy reasons, observations were not undertaken in or directly near the mothers' bedrooms. When occasionally asked by staff, and less often by clients, what we were doing in the MBU, we told them that we were looking at the use of space in the new building. This occasionally resulted in staff or clients giving us direct feedback about an aspect of the MBU. Notes were handwritten during observations, focusing on interactions and movement within the space, and the space itself, and these notes were then subsequently typed up.

Interviews with Architects

Interviews with six architects (five men, one woman) involved in or aligned with the design of the MBU were undertaken by the first author in 2016 and 2018. Architects were asked what they were most satisfied with in the design of the MBU, what the most challenging aspect of designing the MBU was, whether they had received any informal or formal feedback about the design of the MBU, and what evidence base and/or research they draw on for the design of mental health facilities and why. Two individual interviews were conducted in person, one interview was conducted with two architects together in person, and two individual interviews were conducted via telephone due to location. All interviews lasted between thirty and forty minutes.

Interviews with Staff

Interviews were conducted with fifteen unit staff, all of whom were women, and were conducted by the second and first authors. Twelve staff were interviewed individually and three staff were interviewed as a group. In terms of the group interview, staff requested to be interviewed as a group due to the busyness of the nurses' station and their need to be available to continue their work during the interview (including brief absences and attention to babies within the nurses' station). The sharing of information during the group interview provided rich data as staff reminded others of things. The interviews were with a range of staff: nurses, a social worker, a mother-infant therapist, psychologists, psychiatrists, a clinical services coordinator, and a registrar. Staff interviews were conducted in 2016 and 2017, and followed a semi-structured interview schedule, with questions about views on the design, how they think the design of a unit affects their clients' well-being and their own well-being as a worker, how spaces facilitate or inhibit a sense of privacy, and how they think the space facilitates or impedes mother/child relationships and interactions. Interviews took place within the unit and lasted on average for thirty-five minutes.

Interviews with Clients and Family Members

Finally, nine interviews were conducted by the first author with clients and family members (thirteen people in total) in 2017. This included interviews with five mothers individually, one joint interview with one mother and her male partner, one male partner individually, one mother-in-law individually, and a group interview with four mothers. The arrangement of interviews depended on the preferences of the participants and the setting. Mothers interviewed individually were happy to be interviewed alone in an interview room, although two opted for a family member to represent them and also give their own responses. The joint interview with the mother and her partner allowed for the partner to encourage the mother to respond and also to provide emotional support. Finally, the group interview arose as the mothers were all sitting in the dining area with their babies and it would have been disruptive to separate them because they were all chatting and relaxed. The first author suggested those who had given consent could take part in a group interview which was unanimously agreed upon by the mothers. This group interview allowed for discussion between the mothers and support of one another. Interviews focused on four questions: (1) Can we start with you telling me a little about how you find the (designed) space within Park House? (2) What do you think about the privacy at Park House? (3) How do you think this new space helps mother/child relationships and interactions? and (4) Is there anything else you'd like to add about the design and use of space at Park House? Interviews took place within the unit and lasted an average of thirty minutes.

Concluding Thoughts

The existing research indicates that, on the whole, the MBU setting is a favorable environment for interventions and programs which lead to positive outcomes for postpartum mothers who fit the criteria for admission to a psychiatric MBU. However, a notable absence in the sources identified was attention to the built space of MBUs. In fact, we found only one source which explicitly mentioned the physical environment. Wright, Jowsey et al. (2018) briefly discuss the physical environment in their study of experiences of MBUs in New Zealand. They found that participants highly valued comfort and homeliness. The main complaint about the physical environment was noise levels which had negative impacts on sleep. Suggestions for improvement were common, particularly from fathers who participated in the study, with a focus on things such as night lighting, clothing hooks, side tables, exercise facilities, and double beds.

As discussed in chapter 1, research that has focused on the mental health impacts of design more broadly than MBUs clearly indicates that the built space shapes how clients experience mental health units (Connellan et al. 2013) and impacts on mental health outcomes (e.g., Chrysikou 2014). In addition, the majority of existing MBU studies are quantitative in design, although there is a growing tendency to include qualitative approaches that provide a more contextualized picture of the experience of MBUs. It is also evident that more qualitative studies concerning the experiences of staff, clients, partners, and families/visitors in the MBU are needed in order to provide important information concerning the broader contextual information that may influence outcomes for mothers and babies beyond the immediate clinical interventions that they receive, as well as how they experience the space.

This chapter has provided an overview of both the existing research which has been conducted about MBUs and the case study upon which this book is based. This information provides an important contextual background for the rest of the book where we explore the way in which purpose built spaces work in practice and how facilities can be designed to promote positive mental health outcomes.

Chapter 3

The Design

Architect Perspectives

This chapter focuses on the design of mental health facilities from the perspective of philosophical intention. In particular, it focuses on the role of primarily male architects in designing purpose built mental health facilities for mothers and children. This chapter argues that architectural design is a crucial component in the creation of a therapeutic milieu for purpose built mental health facilities, one that needs to be in harmony with the human requirements of the space. It also argues that architects must consider the detailed practical use of specific spaces and the impact of design on mental health outcomes at all stages of the design process. To support this argument, interview data, design briefs/plans, and ethnographic data from the MBU that is the focus of the case study are all drawn upon. Two architecture firms designed the unit; as such, interview data from architects constitute the primary analytic material for the chapter. Pseudonyms are used throughout. Martin, Robert, James, and Derrick are the four principal architects, and Joseph and Louise were aligned to the project. All material referred to is embedded in literature relevant to design, gender, and mental health to provide a broad base.

The MBU that is used as a case study in this book was redesigned a small distance away from the older MBU which was part of a nineteenth-century adult mental health unit situated in parklands. The redevelopment was chiefly because of a state-wide renewal of urban spaces that aimed to maximize their potential with efficient and intelligent design. Although the existing facilities were functional, they needed refurbishment. The MBU was redesigned at the same time as other units with predesign consultations taking approximately four years. Each facility required different types of research and evidence to inform its therapeutic efficacy but all nested together in a section of the original grounds.

The chapter considers the architects' knowledge of evidence relating to the design of mental health facilities, their views on the consultation processes, and reflections on the successes and challenges of the design. These successes and challenges are addressed according to the themes developed from the architects' interview data. The themes include the following: the new model of care; movement through the spaces; internal garden courtyards; safety and privacy; and domesticity. The chapter concludes with a discussion about the need for in-depth consultation and follow-through with users of MBUs, drawing on research evidence relating to the design of mental health facilities for the best psychological outcomes. Design requirements specifically for mothers and babies at that critical stage when a new life joins the world need careful attention with the application of evidence-based research.

EVIDENCE AND DREAMS

"You need a village to raise a child" is an old adage, bringing with it an idealized vision of a community where everyone looks out for each other. This village is an organic whole with dwellings and families linked through trust and tradition. It is a dream. But dreams linger, and unrequited needs within them give rise to creative projects. The garden city, an architectural movement stemming from the late nineteenth-century England is an example of idealized community life that lives on in contemporary residential planning and architecture (Meacham 1999). Isolation is not healthy for anyone and mothers who try raising children without community support tend to have problems. Nonetheless, village communities take generations to shape themselves and develop trust. Can it be proven that a reconstructed village will support mothers and babies who are struggling? We asked the architects what evidence they used.

One firm of architects for Park House has been testing the village concept for mental health facilities for two decades. Martin regarded the twenty years of their work as: "pretty good evidence. It's as good evidence as doing a research paper that's for sure." Robert said they had taken the idea from another mental health project in the north of England and tested it as an urban planning model. He elaborated on the village idea saying:

> You know . . . if you form the village green with the buildings themselves, then again you can . . . go from one building to the next, have a, you know, central shared activity centre from your inpatient wards and back again. And, there isn't that risk of someone either absconding or being vulnerable to other people within a protected ground. . . . And I think unanimously everyone liked the idea

> of the village with the village green that would form a sort of positive focal point for the facility.

The vision of the village and the concept of the internal private garden that Park House was wrapped around were embraced as shared truths. At some point, that dream-vision was validated into acceptable evidence. Martin considered their design of the secure internal garden for an MBU as having had an "impact" because it had been adopted by other architects in various countries. This is an example of practice-based evidence in design.

However there is no real consensus for what constitutes evidence in architecture and particularly for the design of MBUs. The editors of a special issue on evidence in architecture write: "How and why is architecture, as a field of knowledge, extended into other and possibly multiple domains of 'truth?'" (Leach, Taylor, and Stickells 2013, 1). An MBU "institution" is one domain of truth (Rose 1999, 2). Martin and Robert promoted truths based on their architectural, and therefore empirical, experience. According to Leach, Taylor, and Stickells (2013, 4), architectural evidence can be divided into three types: "procedural" which includes the documented process of how the building(s) came about; "contextual" which includes the agencies of all involved as well as unexpected aspects; and "conceptual" such as architectural drawings. These three categories are not neatly circumscribed, and when it comes to large mental health projects such as the one Park House sits in, health departments require quantitative data and "scientific truth" (Rose 1998, 72).

Evidence-based medicine and evidence-based health design are not necessarily worlds apart; both can learn from each other because responses to the built environment can affect pain and anxiety (McLaughlan 2017). There are, however, blind spots for evidence in medicine just as there are blind spots for evidence in architecture, but crucially, as Redhouse (2019) notes, a lack of evidence does not necessarily mean that the area with more evidence is the route to follow. As a mother who experienced the panic of being a first, and then second time mother, Redhouse (2019) writes of her resistance to the scientific determinism of diagnostic tools. As such the contextual evidence gathered from listening (interviews), observing (ethnographies), and evaluating these data can augment both the fields of psychiatric and architectural research.

Procedural evidence in architecture is the most complex as there are multiple models for documenting and evaluating architectural projects and they demand financial investment which is rarely provided (Connellan et al. 2013; Edwards 2011; Golembiewski 2010; International Living Future Institute 2019; Stichler 2008). James, an architect from the second firm involved with Park House bemoaned the absence of procedural evidence with regard to mental health facility design, saying that it "makes a mockery of the whole process." James added, "We did do quite a lot of research and struggled to find any real evidence to support what we were doing." Most of the architects noted the prevalence of anecdotal information and James specifically asked "how do you measure success [in the design of a mental health unit]?" James pointed out the lack of continuity in gathering information while they were working on Park House and the other units around it, saying that when it came to handover stage, the project management group who had been part of the consultation phase were no longer in existence and the facility management took over. He added, "They had no history . . . didn't refer back to the original documents for principles" with different divisions and services running independently from each other. James cited an example of a children's hospital in Melbourne where funding for tracking progress and gathering data was built into the whole project from its earliest consultation phase. In this way research for procedural evidence was intrinsic, with specific people assigned to follow changes throughout the project and provide essential continuity. This type of procedural evidence is ideally captured in reviews that systematically compare original briefs with actual outcomes at post occupancy. This process closes the consultation, handover, pre and post occupancy feedback loop, taking lessons from previous projects (Connellan et al. 2013). There are several terms and models for evaluations and reviews of buildings which come from the diverse disciplines involved, each with its own language and vision (Pearce 2018). This brings us to the next topic in the lead-up to the design for Park House: the consultation and briefing phase.

CONSULTATION: PARALLEL DEMOCRACIES

Democratic processes of listening, talking, including, and respecting may be understood at one level but at ground level they can falter. Writing on the politics of design, Tony Fry (2011, 34) claims that democracy is fractured, filled with rhetoric, and "the people . . . are an absent signifier." Consultations for redevelopment and design of Park House commenced eight years prior to completion. These consultations had a legal responsibility to include all stakeholder representatives, that is crucial people connected with the site past and present. The site is that of an old asylum-style campus situated in approximately thirty hectares of parkland. Phases one and two of the Master Plan were based on an urban village with shared green spaces sensitively landscaped into the park with its established trees and heritage buildings. Written objections to the proposals for land clearance, as well as the absence of engagement with Indigenous representatives, were not taken on board. Historic buildings were sold to corporations and land clearance took place before any residential and road approvals were granted; as a result, eighty-three significant trees were cut down. The "pluralism" required to ensure democratic consultation processes actually worked was not enacted (Fry 2011, 35). The following paragraphs draw from masterplans, briefs, reports, and policy documents which are standard for a new public health facility (note that we have not directly referenced these documents as they identify the hospital, MBU, its staff, and the architects).

The specific design briefing consultations included topics such as the need for a homelike domestic environment that was located within the local community or at least close enough to facilitate reintegration. The environment was to be: filled with natural light; welcoming; calm; safe and private; and provide "multidisciplinary holistic biopsychosocial rehabilitation" services. The basic concept was to maintain a domestic layout and promote a sense of continuity with everyday life. The character of the designs was to be reassuring and noninstitutional with a pleasant atmosphere while retaining necessary functional requirements, including robust materials and furnishings. Simple, quiet, but shared, living areas were recommended with views of the outside gardens regarded as essential and direct access to them as desirable. These gardens were to be carefully landscaped affording a sensitive and nurturing environment. The design was expected to anticipate the clients' needs for independence and dignity, while simultaneously enabling staff to supervise and observe. To this end security was to be unobtrusive but protective of staff and clients especially at night. Ease of movement and avoidance of congestion was an imperative and with this came the first challenges for the smaller spaces in the new build. Hospital design typically avoids "undue contact, contagion, physical proximity and overcrowding" (Foucault 1980, 146). Flexibility of spatial design with open planning and interchangeable use of some areas were therefore an early consideration.

The consultations did not proceed smoothly. Interactions in the consultation phase are necessarily "constituted by difference and conflict," which can be a productive aspect in a democratic process, unless they run in parallel worlds without adequate understanding, compromise, and resolution (Massey 1994, 139). The initial planning process which led to the crucial Specialist Health Services Design Brief and Master Plan was beset with contesting opinions. Neither the staff from the existing MBU nor the architects felt they were being heard. Robert commented that there were a "very large number of strong personalities within this user group [Park House] who were not open to discussing new ideas. Too many cooks . . . [un]representative of all the users." This issue of inadequate representation emerged as significant later when the design was already underway.

Design briefing specific to Park House constituted 7 pages of the 165-page Design Brief. It described the scope for a specialist perinatal and infant mental health service, across obstetrics, inpatient, outpatient, and community. Service aims in the brief stipulated the promotion of robust mental health at the very earliest opportunity for future generations, intervention in the life cycle, and preservation of the mother-baby relationship together with families while developing independence. James and Derrick, in separate interviews, noted that based on their experience of other project briefs, the brief for the whole mental health hospital was "very, very restrictive" and "very detailed and very demanding and very specific, particularly about what was close to what."

The staff, who were predominantly women, voiced concern about placing young women and children beside other adult mental health units. James and Derrick identified a particular woman clinician as being "very passionate" and "intense." From the architects' perspective, this intensity came from women clinicians stressing the vulnerability of people in Park House and the "potential threats" from clients in "adjacent units."

The architects reported finding the consultations regarding Park House more difficult than consultations with other units, with James saying that the staff in another unit within the same hospital precinct was "a dream client" and "just absolutely beautiful to work with." However, both James and Derrick acknowledged that the culture of Park House was different to other units and that there were more challenges involved for staff of Park House because a "new model of care was being imposed on them" alongside the new facilities. Working with the health professionals was claimed as "one of the most challenging aspects," with James saying "for a group of people that are there to care for probably the most sick in society, um, the things that they can say and the mental stress that they can put you under themselves, is probably far from what you would expect from a health clinician." This discomfort was apparently felt more keenly by the architects in the consultation stage, because after the above quoted statement, James added that when the clinicians from Park House came onto the building site, "they were actually quite lovely most of the time."

There were fewer women architects involved in the consultations than there were women health representatives. Martin referred to only one woman architect being part of the consultations, but she was not interviewed; Martin said that he was representing what others (including that woman architect) had shared with him prior to the interview because the interview questions were available to all of them. Louise, an architect who *was* interviewed, and was on the staff of one of the architectural firms at the time of the Park House design did not comment on the consultations because she had not been part of that initial phase. Louise's comments are included in the next subsection. It is worth noting that both architecture firms are large and not everyone connected with the project took part in the consultations. Additionally, the staff of the architecture firms did not remain the same, for example, when the authors tried to find the woman architect who had been part of the consultations she had left the firm.

SUCCESSES AND CHALLENGES OF DESIGNS

The issues with consultation spilled over into the design. Six themes that speak to the successes and challenges emerged from an analysis of the architect interview data include the following: the old mortuary, model of care, movement, gardens, safety/privacy, and domesticity. These are covered in that order below. While the focus will be on the data from the architects, at times when there is a crossover, the discussion will include data from staff, patients/families, and ethnographic observations.

The Old Mortuary

Agrest (2000, 358) writes that "[s]omewhere every culture has an imaginary zone for what it excludes, and it is this zone that we must try to remember today." The cycle of life and death within ancestral country is circular and those who have passed are not gone, they remain to provide guidance and their spirits linger in their places of passing (Hafner 2013). This poignancy is elaborated upon below in the discussion of an old mortuary building on the site of Park House.

A stand out feature that was under addressed in the consultation phase for Park House, and which created a significant stumbling block in the design phase, was the old mortuary. This building is a small neo-Gothic heritage-listed building on the precise site where Park House was to be built. In the days of the old asylum-styled facility it was annotated as "The Dead House" and was where autopsies took place in addition to laying out the deceased prior to burial. It has the heading "The Old Morgue" in the design brief, but only six sentences are devoted to it, with no clarity regarding its reuse.

The senior architects directly involved in the design wanted the old mortuary building to be repurposed as an entrance for Park House, thereby forming a front of house that was unique from the other units. Martin saw it as "quite a nice little pavilion [that would] make a very simple entry porch." "Pavilion" in architectural terminology is both a structural and decorative space used for displaying, viewing, and performing. The pavilion is a commonly used term in large international art and architectural exhibitions. It is used to designate a particular country's or city's exhibit and came into everyday usage during the nineteenth-century age of large-scale expositions of national pride (Adams 2005). In terms of the old mortuary on the site of Park House, the architects "embraced it" as a courtyard portal into Park House, despite the operational need for an inpatient and outpatient entrance, saying that "we've managed that as well." This design idea developed right into the design phase and the rest of Park House was oriented toward its north facing prospect.

The architectural heritage of the mortuary building was understood and, as stated above, "embraced" by the architects, but the sensitive indigenous and cultural heritage did not receive the same attention. Objections to the mortuary as an entrance "had not been not been taken on board" in the consultation phase. Sally, a senior staff member noted that there was a "lack of Indigenous consultation from the very beginning [and] months after initial planning" when Indigenous Australians were invited in the planning process, "they said they would not use it because of cultural prohibition." Failure to engage appropriately with the local Indigenous people contravened the Master Plan which stated quite clearly that consultation with the original custodians of the land would take place *before* any redevelopment occurred on site.

At that late stage the design for Park House, which was in a figure of 8 with the mortuary on the front loop, could not be changed. "Cultural prohibition" put an immediate stop to the incorporation and reuse of the mortuary into Park House. The result was that the mortuary building remains but it is inaccessible with only façades visible (see figure 3.1).

The Masterplan stated that, in accordance with law, a cultural heritage survey was "being" undertaken, but that a search of the "Register of Aboriginal Sites and Objects" indicated there were no "known entries" on the site of the old asylum-style campus. When asked about Indigenous representation in a follow-up question during one of the architect interviews, that architect said: "I'm not familiar enough with the local group [of Indigenous people] . . . I would expect so. The major projects team from the State Health department were very thorough in organising consultation with the community so I would imagine so but I can't say yes or no."

As mentioned previously, up to this point all the architects who were interviewed and who voiced their willingness to use the mortuary as an entrance were men. At a later date the authors of this book wanted to explore gender and architecture more closely, and it became obvious that the architects involved in the design were primarily men. The absence of women architect voices was clear, and additional ethics clearance to interview women architects was obtained to address the gap. The first issue that arose in an interview with Louise, an architect aligned with the project, was that of the mortuary. Louise questioned the sense of putting mothers, some of whom were at acute risk of harming themselves and/or their babies, adjacent to an old mortuary. When she was asked if she voiced her concerns to the other architects at the time, she replied, "I did, but the decisions were so far down the track, nothing

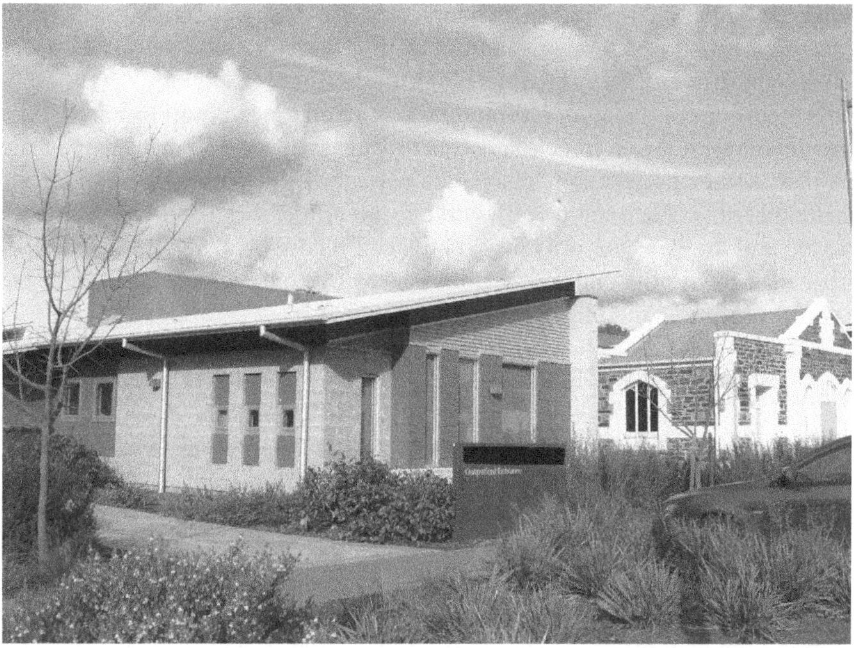

Figure 3.1 Outpatient Entrance Showing Historic Mortuary Building. *Source*: Photographed by Kathleen Connellan.

I said could change it." The data from this interview are worth quoting more fully as it throws light on gender issues alongside the topic of the mortuary:

Interviewer: How were your comments received?
Louise: Ah there might have been some raised eyebrows, I might have been very selective who I said that to, I worked out there was quite a bit of hierarchy within the whole set up, so I realised that nothing I said would make any . . . well you couldn't make any changes because all the planning approvals had gone through, . . . and possibly even concrete had been poured for the site . . . .
Interviewer: Okay . . . so you remember whether it was being used as the entrance?
Louise: Yes I do and I remember being absolutely gobsmacked at having to . . . enter a mental health unit, and I feel myself getting quite angry about this, why on earth would you put the entry to a mental health facility through a mortuary? It's not like you, . . . if it's heritage you have to retain the name, "Old Mortuary," so it's not like you can kind of whitewash the purpose of that building.

The above perspective is specific to the plight of women and their mental proximity to loss and grief associated with their babies. Some women would recall miscarriages, still births, and other instances of losing a child; in this way, death and birth are closely aligned. Even in "developed" countries it is relatively recent that giving birth guarantees life. Many countries still experience high infant and mother fatalities during the vulnerable perinatal stages (Roser and Ritchie 2019; Wagstaff 2000).

The concept of using an old mortuary as an entrance portal to Park House was abandoned; the architects subsequently changed the entrance design from a single entrance foyer to two separate entrances: one for inpatients and one for outpatients. Each entrance is around the corner from the Old Mortuary façade and they are not obviously entrances. These changes presented challenges for the north/south orientation that was to maximize natural light but also for reception and movement in the new model of care.

Model of Care

The change to a model of care that champions integration of mind, body, and community, and is shared by an interdisciplinary team of experts, contrasted with the previously less integrated model and it was not immediately simple to implement. From some of the architects' perspectives, there was a view that staff in other units understood and accepted the change more than the staff of Park House. Consequently, change management was integral to adapting the new model of care to the new spatial design of Park House for health administration and architects. Martin said they were determined to "invert how the original asylum worked" and not have "the staff . . . creating a monster. We wanted to try and break that down." Martin admitted he was not sure that this was "the role of the architect" but said that new integrated approaches to care also demanded integrated spatial arrangements.

The changes demanded upgraded technologies for advanced ways of working with and monitoring mothers and babies. The architects noted that the budget for these changes was a concern "all the way through" and "a lot of the funding for change management [including technology] was definitely cut." The principal architects were disappointed that their vision could not be fully realized as a result of compromise and budgetary constraints. Robert noted that environmental factors and user needs will always change and future proofing is required wherever possible, but in the design of mental health facilities, change is seen "at a tragic level." By this, Robert pointed to the emotionally charged atmosphere in mental health facilities given the vulnerabilities of the clients.

In a guided walk-through of the previous MBU, a mental health nurse commented personally to [author 1] that "mental health nurses have long memories" (May 28, 2010). These were memories of violent attacks upon nurses and doctors by patients; such narratives perpetuated a culture of fear which lay just beneath the surface of staff with particularly long tenures at the facility. These staff members wanted clear lines of sight but also sufficient separate and dedicated rooms for privacy and safety in the new facility. However, as discussed in chapter 5, many staff members welcomed the new design with open flexible spaces.

During the building construction period some of the old facilities were refitted to "test some of the [new] model of care principles" and to facilitate the move from old to new spaces. Park House was included in that trial but according to two architects, not all the staff took up the opportunity for a change in their practice. The architects noted that there were "teething problems" but also that some staff in Park House were "early-adopters" of that style of interactive staffing. Robert's perception was that the staff were "dominant" and had "not been properly change managed." However, as chapter 5 shows, Park House staff are not a homogenous group. There is already contradictory data from the architects who in one instance claim that Park House had the new care plan "imposed upon them" and in another that they were "early-adopters" of it given the nature of their work with the babies.

A key spatial issue in the change of care was the placement, size, and function of the nurses' station in Park House. Previously the nurses' station had provided clear lines of sight and, according to some staff, also provided ample work space. Therefore, in that design scenario, the staff who wanted to could remain in the nurses' station for longer and could still observe the mothers reasonably clearly. The nurses' station was one of the main features the architects wanted to decentralize, and they did this by situating it off to one side, reducing its floor space (3,510 m × 5,250 m) and glazing on two sides only. The intention was to discourage long stays, restrict the amount of administrative work that could be done, and ensure that the nurses' station did not operate like a panopticon: "so that it's not the central thing that everything circulates around" (see figure 3.2).

The architects said that the nurses' station in Park House was "probably the most secure of all the staff stations" in the whole of the hospital complex. It was not designed for patients to approach and converse with staff, it does not have opening glass panels, and the door is supposed to be kept closed at all times. It was also certainly not designed as a clinical space or to accommodate babies. The nurses' station is perhaps the clearest example of a breakdown in functionality. As we found in our observations, it was often a "chaotic" space, with sometimes eight staff in there at one time. Below is an excerpt from the ethnographic data taken between 12.14 p.m. and 12.16 p.m. on a weekday:

> It's very hectic in here and not enough chairs for nurses to sit on. Man [nurse] is using computer and I have his chair. . . . Staff are moving in and out too quickly for me to count and track their movements. Door is now unlocked and wide open. Mental health nurse brings in baby in stroller, parks stroller in middle of

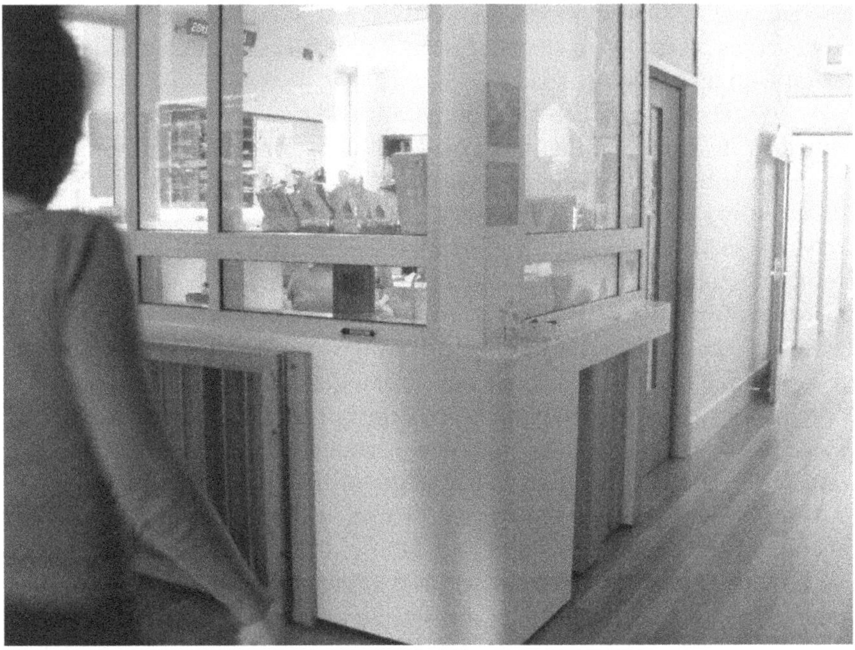

Figure 3.2 Nurses' Station Exterior. *Source*: Photographed by Kathleen Connellan.

the office—it's a very small space for multiple staff members let alone a stroller too.

Staff brought babies in prams into the nurses' station when the nurseries were full, or when they needed to continue to observe them. With a floor space of 18.2 square meters and only four office chairs assigned to the space, it is a prime example of the disjuncture between the architects' perception of the new model of care and the staff uptake of it (see figures 3.3 and 3.4). Storage for the staff's personal items (including their packed lunches) in the inpatient unit is located in the staff toilets which staff objected to, therefore the nurses' station tended to be cluttered with many items including bags.

The nurses' station originally had a dividing panel to section off a smaller administrative area with surveillance monitors and bedroom audio receptors but that panel was later partially removed leaving a section protruding into the space and interfering with movement and causing one nurse to trip during our ethnographic observations. Joseph noted his partner architect in the firm "had a deep passion . . . for removing staff stations" altogether. Joseph's idea is that the nurses' station is just a small administrative base and nurses should continually interact with mothers and babies in line with the new model of patient-centered integrated care.

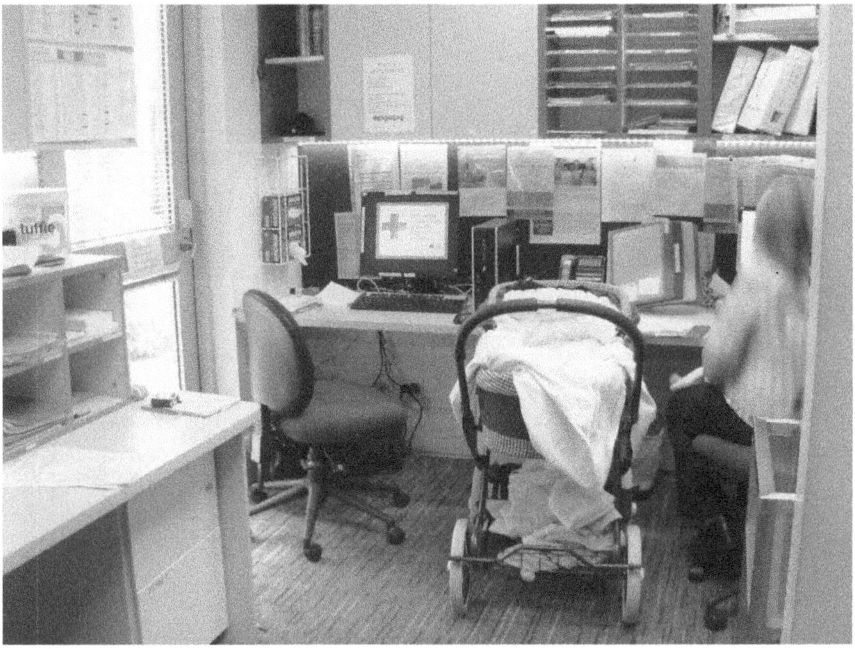

Figure 3.3 Nurses' Station Interior. *Source*: Photographed by Kathleen Connellan.

The architects intended most administration as well as staff relaxation to be done in an entirely different building which necessitated leaving Park House and walking outdoors. The architects were disappointed to hear that those staff facilities were underutilized. These issues that are related to staff activity link to the larger concept of movement which is another important theme from the architects' data.

Movement

Flowing, open architectural design encourages and determines movement through and into spaces. The design of Park House is a fluid figure of eight around two secure internal garden courtyards. The architects wanted to create dynamic spaces throughout so that the static nature of older models of care could not work. The floor plan of Park House (see figure 3.5) is consequently not based on a conventional grid with the linear corridors typical of older hospitals.

Architects consciously opened out the previous essentialism of demarcated spaces with their territorial and directional signage; Martin in particular was emphatically against named spaces. Martin stressed that they wanted casual and clinical interactions to occur as people passed by and paused to talk. As

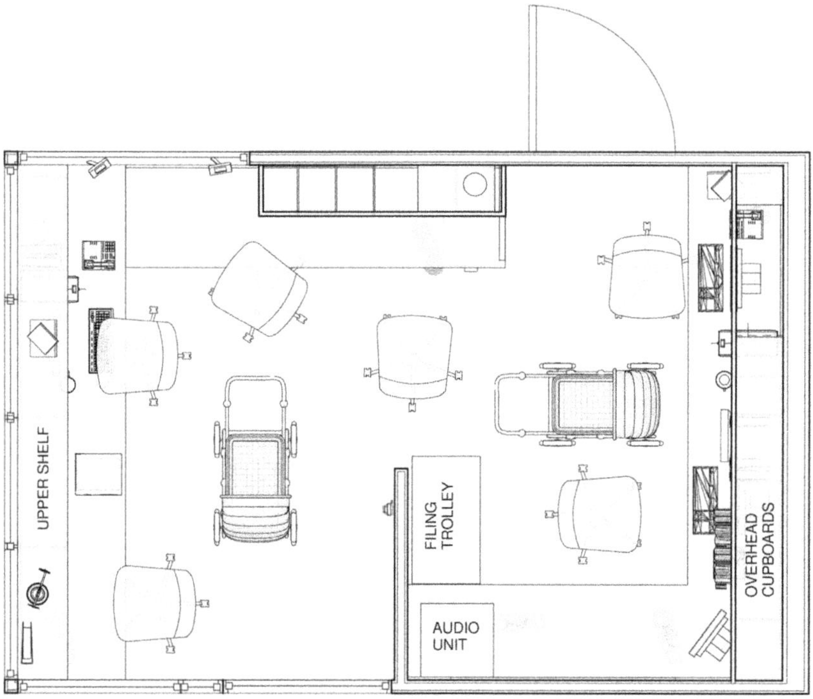

Figure 3.4 Nurses' Station Showing Furniture and Prams. *Source*: Image drawn by Roxanne Adams for Kathleen Connellan.

such, the spaces were designed to invite a loose type of movement encouraging social exchange without being obviously clinical. Martin noted:

> We had to think of ways of subverting the default position by . . . instead of designing the building . . . as an insurance policy, so—the panopticon approach [which] is like having an insurance against all the things that can go wrong, what we thought was, well why don't we design the building so that [it] can become an insurance policy but [yet] allow positive things to happen, rather than negative things.

By this Martin meant they designed a space that did ensure safety, but that kind of "insurance" was not the sole objective. It was also important to channel movement to permit worthwhile exchanges, as mentioned above. For example, staff, including the psychiatrists who have offices in the outpatient section, needed to walk through a large, light, open, multipurpose dining space with several round tables and chairs on their way to the nurses' station. It is not the only way but it is the most direct route and as a result it is used

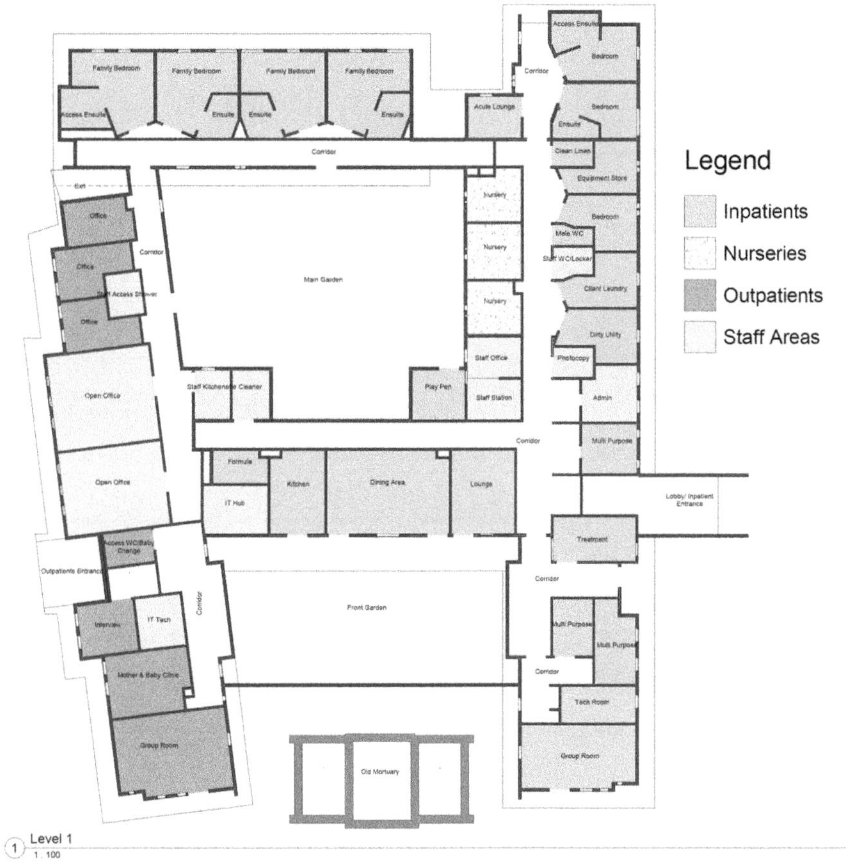

Figure 3.5 Spatial Allocation Plan. *Source*: Drawn by Roxanne Adams for Kathleen Connellan.

as a thoroughfare by staff. In line with the architects' intentions staff were mobile and did not remain in the nurses' station or offices for long periods of time. Observational data show movement to be lively and frequent during the day with less at night (overall the word "walk" comes up 195 times in our transcribed ethnographic data, covering both staff and clients). This was the design intention that actively enhanced the new model of care; therefore facilitating conversations with clients sitting in the dining area reading, doing art/craft work, having a snack, or just being with their babies. Most mothers and staff welcomed the informal interaction in communal spaces, although some did have misgivings about privacy if the conversation became clinical and a private space was not available.

The architectural control of movement through space also affected the mothers who had to leave their bedrooms, walk past the nurses' station,

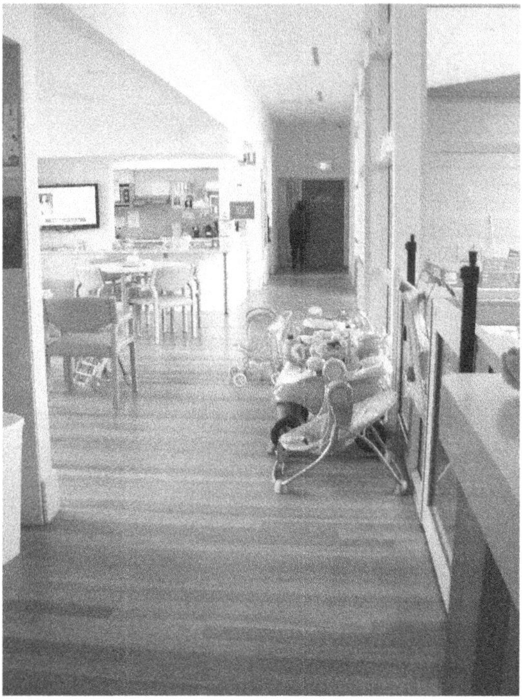

Figure 3.6 Part of the Route to the Formula Room. *Source*: Photographed by Kathleen Connellan.

through the dining area to eventually arrive at the formula room to prepare their baby's milk bottle or at the kitchen to prepare a snack (see figure 3.6). This encouraged the mothers to interact with other mothers or nurses if any were passed on the way. One grandmother we interviewed commented,

> It actually forces her to interact with people, because she actually has to leave her bedroom to get everything because it's away from the room so I don't know whether that's been purposely done because sometimes when you're depressed you want to shut yourself away so as much as sometimes it's a pain having to come all the way all around to get the formula. I think sometimes that it's been done on purpose because in the process you get to see different people on the way around and interact with people.

The positive aspects of coming together in shared spaces was also felt at a research level because an impromptu group interview was conducted with consenting mothers who all just happened to be sitting with their babies in the dining area at the same time; as such, it was more natural as well as less disruptive to engage with them together. The same thing happened in the nurses' station, although it was cramped.

The design strategy and realization of movement were both a "success" and a challenge. Success in health design must necessarily be linked to evidence, and as explained previously in this chapter, "evidence" remains highly contingent. The movement of both staff and clients was designed into the space with staff movement disguised to appear less determined. Mothers, on the other hand, tended to move through the spaces more slowly, however when the destination was fixed (such as the baby formula room) there also tended to be a purposefulness to their movement.

Gardens

The gardens in Park House are a key design feature for the new model of care, with the intention of encouraging interaction for the mothers, babies/toddlers, and families. The unit is literally wrapped around two central gardens; each garden is designed as an inviting nucleus with its open sky, sunlight, fresh air, blend of soft lines, greenery, and play equipment. The bedroom windows look out onto the exterior gardens of the larger hospital, but the walkways and open-plan spaces in Park House look out to the internal gardens. Both internal gardens are accessible for the inpatients with the larger one exclusively for inpatient use (see figure 3.7). The larger garden is a space where families meet on a Friday afternoon for a barbecue picnic; adequate facilities ensure the informality of this casual get together. The outdoor furnishings echo an Australian backyard that is carefully tended but consciously designed for young children with the play equipment dominating the area.

The gardens are not shared with other units so mothers and babies can feel secure and not in the company of differently unwell people. The architects' idea was "to embed the gardens in the middle of these units because perimeter gardens . . . require more trust, more independence, and if you like—less ability to observe." The architects were restricted by the amount of land available and could not incorporate a garden to "get lost in," which is what Joseph believes in. Joseph added, "The idea of getting lost in a psychiatric facility garden here in Australia would be just completely dismissed because everywhere there has to be observation." Mental health research invoking nature, gardens, and fresh air as an essential design component that is integral to healing almost always reminisces upon the large grounds of the nineteenth-century asylums. The change in models of care since the asylum model included the loss of those expansive landscaped grounds (Chrysikou 2014; Hickmann 2009).

Visibility is a complex issue in mental health and will be discussed in more detail in the next subsection on safety and privacy, but in terms of the internal

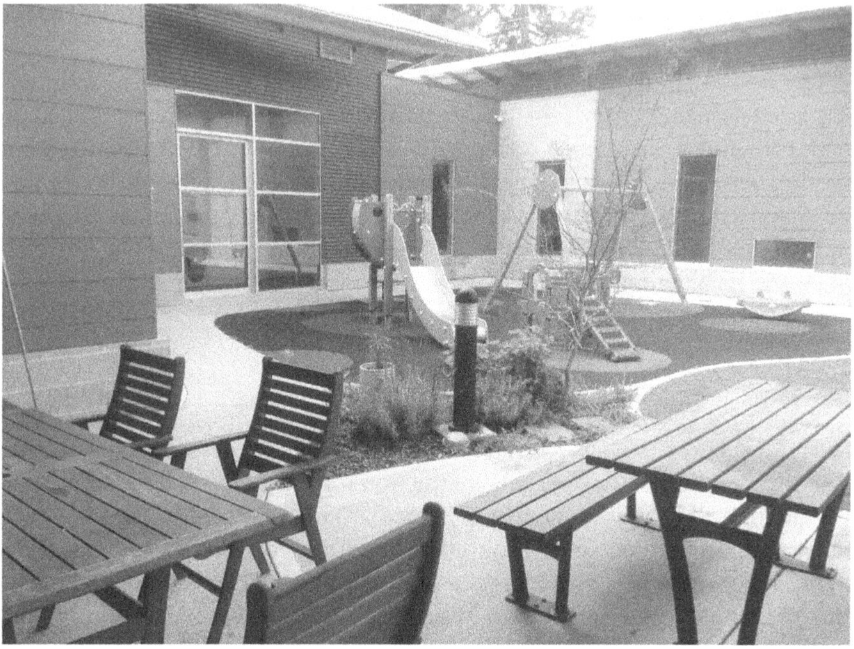

Figure 3.7 Main Garden Showing Picnic Tables/Area. *Source*: Photographed by Kathleen Connellan.

gardens which are glazed on four sides, the nurses can see the mothers and babies and mothers can also see into the gardens. The garden is a panopticon without having the effect of being so; the data do not distinctly indicate that when people are in the garden they feel particularly observed, however as researchers sitting in the space we felt conspicuous. In the absence of private consultation/interview room availability, mothers could also go outside to extend conversations that may have commenced in the dining area but which required more sound privacy.

Joseph believes in the salutogenic approach where "a patient actually goes and touches a tree" and where elements of surprise, adventure, and discovery are endlessly available in a natural garden setting (Golembiewski 2010). This approach shares some aspects with the Planetree method, which is reputedly named after the tree under which Hippocrates taught his students (Stichler 2008). Planetree, like Salutogenics, is patient-centered and focuses upon healing interactions (Stichler 2008). Joseph is an architect keenly aware of the need for research across mental health outcomes and nature. However, he voiced criticism regarding the "blind spot" in gardens and architecture for mental health and, as with Connellan, Due, and Riggs (2015), Joseph believes that if gardens are designed to be looked through "impenetrable walls of glass" there is a deceit in the design which is unfair to patients in the unit. Joseph added, "Under those circumstances [patients can see but not go into the garden] I believe that nature is a poison" because it pretends to be available, yet its affordances are denied. Indeed, a key element in building the mother–baby relationship is availability; being visible but unavailable is detrimental to building healthy attachments. The paragraph below outlines problems of garden accessibility which impedes the effectiveness of the central and "available" garden in Park House.

A garden is, among other things, a place to play in. Play therapy is part of the suite of interventions used by clinicians to enhance attachment in formal therapy sessions, however informal play is also extremely valuable (Bilszta et al. 2012). Toddlers especially need space to run around, explore, and experiment; but unfortunately the functional interior design/exterior flow of space into the garden does not work in Park House. If toddlers in the unit wanted to venture out into the garden space through the large sliding doors from the dining area, they could not because the doors have to be kept closed on account of the air conditioning system.

The air conditioning is centrally controlled and will malfunction if outside air interferes with the temperature setting. This was disappointing for the architects who had intended for a natural and relatively unimpeded flow in and out of the large internal garden from the dining area. It was also frustrating for the nurses and the mothers, many of whom complained about the lack of fresh air in the unit. Unfortunately, the fresh air from both internal and exterior gardens could not permeate the building. Bedroom windows could not open and the effect of constant air conditioning was unpleasant. Therefore, in a room where a mother may be at her lowest ebb, nature's freshness was restricted to a semblance.

Nonetheless, the glassed garden spaces are bright centers in the ambience of Park House but at times the nurses in particular found that the light was too harsh and they said the blinds over the dining area (as well as elsewhere) were difficult to operate. Natural light is essential in a healing environment and the architects were determined to maximize its potential (Connellan et al. 2013; Anjali et al. 2016; Stichler 2009; Ulrich 2008). The idea was to minimize the use of artificial lighting as much as possible. The architects wanted the circadian rhythms of nature to permeate the buildings and in a general comment Martin said, "The beauty about these buildings is if you walk around even at dusk, often you find the lights are not turned on." The observational data have multiple references to the natural light flooding into the spaces during the day and, despite the wintery time of the year, artificial lights were rarely on in the dining area.

Safety/Privacy

Park House with its vulnerable young women and children requires particular shielding from the other mental health units so that mothers can feel safe and private. The internal gardens are a design solution for creating an exterior within an interior so that the unit does not resemble a "category B prison." Robert said that they wanted to ensure "privacy and dignity in terms of people using the facility having ready access to outside space, the building itself being welcoming as opposed to intimidating." However, there was a feeling that the architects could not go as far as they wanted to in terms of the relationship between the indoors and the outdoors: "I think we could have gone further . . . but it all gets a little bit lost in translation when you have user groups . . . who've got a focus on security." Martin noted that if "you've got safety and security problems in a unit, it's either going to be because the regime is so repressive or oppressive." The perception among the architects was that the nurses were concerned for their own safety, in a comment that seemed to refer to the design across all units, Joseph noted: "And you know they trotted out all the same excuses that you hear every day, about, you know, the nurses' safety, and the nurses this and the nurses that. Never mind the fact that the place was always compromised by its location [on the historic asylum-style site]."

Our observations as well as client and staff interviews do not reveal any specific details about the nurses' safety; on the contrary, the data reveal greater concerns for the mothers' and babies' safety. This was particularly obvious in relation to mothers going out for a smoke at nighttime outside the building (not in enclosed garden spaces), which is a topic that is covered in chapter 5 "The Workspace: Staff Perspectives." Additionally, our observations note that the entrance door for the inpatients at Park House was left unlocked at times.

Privacy, conversely, was an issue for all groups. For the architects it was about disguising the institutional and panoptic effects of surveillance. For the staff it was about confidentiality during counseling which, as discussed earlier, took place at impromptu times. The staff felt there were insufficient rooms but the architects wanted to move away from rows of "rooms" to an open-plan which offered clients a few spots to sit without feeling watched. Architects wanted to make those places seem as natural as possible. The gardens, loosely arranged dining space, and entrance lobby which looked out onto the smaller garden offered many opportunities to pause with degrees of privacy.

Privacy was linked to noise for the mothers, the doors to their bedrooms had hand towels looped over the doors so that they would not bang and disturb sleep, but this also meant that they were often left ajar which compromised the mother's privacy. Doors can be designed to close quietly but there was obviously an issue with door noises in Park House, as our notes show: "A door I can't see near the other kitchen on the left is opened and closed several times, it's loud and jarring, a heavy door that keeps loudly clicking closed." It was also possible to hear noises through internal walls; one mother complained that she could hear "crying, crying," through the walls and said "you have to make a design that's quieter . . . and space . . . to have a little bit privacy, privacy." A grandmother interviewed and three other mothers saw the benefit of having to leave the bedroom for most things and considered the balance between privacy and security adequate.

Domesticity

The title of this book *Home and Away: Mothers and Babies in Institutional Spaces* holds domesticity at its heart. Domesticity, or more precisely domesticities, comprise(s) a mixture of meanings. The architects wanted to create a "residential, domestic feeling . . . in a much more interesting way [than the institutional mental hospital]." As explained in chapter 1: Introduction, home and motherhood are historically connected through cultural constructions of home. Park House is both home and institution and the challenge for architects and interior architects was to reinterpret both using best practice design principles. Best practice is synonymous with "good design" (Hayward 1998), which is an approach that stems from modernist design principles where efficiency and high quality materials come together. When "good design" is combined with notions of "good home," "good mother," and "good baby" there is a pyramid of expectations with good mother at the pinnacle.

Against the above ideals, the architects were nonetheless at pains to produce a home that incorporated the "usual" spaces in a contemporary suburban family home. In this way there was an attempt to incorporate the best of modernist architectural principles with more relaxed and flexible postmodern approaches. These include a light filled open-plan living/dining/kitchen area opening out onto a back garden with an entertainment area, a separate lounge and television room, and bedrooms with en suite bathrooms. This is precisely what Park House has, *but* it also has much more. It is these extra (clinical and administrative) spaces that the architects wanted to disguise or decentralize. Apart from the open-plan approach, separate rooms in the inpatient section that were not part of the domestic arrangement were given generic names as a disguise but also so that they could be multipurposed. Martin used the term "deception" to explain the conscious design departure from blatantly obvious mental health design. Martin felt that it was necessary to suspend the literal realities of being "fenced" off from the outside world in a way that was less confronting for the mothers. MBUs such as Park House mirror domestic architecture as part of a crucial de-stigmatization from what Adrian Forty (1984) calls the indelible link between madness and its built form.

The inpatient section of Park House which is the focus of this book cannot be divorced from the design of the whole because this is what is seen from the outside. It is a home in a larger mental health "institution," it is a home linked to an outpatients' section that has the clinicians' offices, therapy, and conference rooms; that is the reality but the ambience is not institutional from the architects or the staff and clients' point of view. The "intimate scale of the spaces" is what contributes to the domestic as opposed to institutional feel according to Martin. However, the small scale was also considered restrictive and cramped by staff and some clients.

The interior design of Park House is where design details including furnishings contribute to a homelike environment. Nonetheless, regulations on risk presented restrictions. A senior architect commented: "The thing I find really ghastly when I would go in there, were the bloody cots! . . . They were like little prisons!" He added that he found some of "the paraphernalia" difficult and the furniture "very institutional." Comparing the Park House interior to examples he had been "uplifted" by in Denmark (Chousein 2015), and referring to the bedrooms, this architect continued to say: "If you go into a unit like this in Denmark, it'll have a pendant light hanging down, there'll be a Poulson lamp, you know, there'll be probably a trolley with china on it, and a flask of coffee, there'll be proper cutlery."

The vignette described by this architect is markedly different to Park House which has a transient functionalism more in line with short stays than a place to feel at home in. However, as Louise noted, the design does provide visual and tactile interest to an otherwise institutional sameness with material combinations of brick, corrugated iron, color bond cladding, and brick cladding.

As mentioned earlier, there were two architecture firms responsible for Park House and one was more involved with the interior design than the other. The division of work is "clearly split" between the "envelope of the building," which falls entirely with the architects, and the interiors, which falls entirely with the interior designers and interior architects. Louise provided more information on the interior design detailing of Park House because she assisted in training the interior designers in a new software program that translates 2-D designs to 3-D, adding that this software is "very unkind to detailed objects such as joinery." This is an important consideration for domesticity concerns within interior design because such software design contributes to a uniformity that can easily be construed as institutional sameness. This then reinforces normative neutralities unless they are balanced with more uniquely designed finishes. The staff in the interior department had to simultaneously learn this new software while designing the details for Park House. Interestingly, the staff in the interior department were all women.

These women were referred to as "the girls" by the male architects. Louise said she pulled the men up on this:

> I picked them up once or twice about that and I said they are "women" but it was always "the girls." And we're talking about women here who ranged from new graduates all the way up well into their forties, and in fact one of the associates [in the firm] was an interior [architect] and probably in her late thirties or early forties, and so the narrative was they were the girls and they were having a hard time with the new [software] programme.

Most women architects prefer to be known simply as architects and not have "woman" or "female" as a prefix in their profession (Walker 2000); this is also the case for interior architects and designers. However, the gender divide between those responsible for the structure and those responsible for interior design is universally known. No interior architects were interviewed or suggested for interviewing by the architectural firms. The data from interviews with architects reveal that there was some dissatisfaction with the interior architects' choice of some furnishing, finishes, and detailing. An excerpt worth quoting is: "And you know we end up in these places choosing all this weird stuff which doesn't look very domestic. Um, I also found a cage I think in one of the rooms . . . was it the kitchen or the dining room . . . a sort of bloody, there's a cage around part of the room!"

This "cage" is the play pen for older babies and toddlers in the dining area below the nurses' station interior window, and is filled with toys (see figure 3.8). The data from the staff and mothers in the unit also reveal dissatisfaction with the design of this play section. Their feeling was that it was far too small to be functional. The play pen is a good example of colliding object–subject relations in the material culture of Park House. Colorful and enticing toys sat together in the pen but the space they inhabited did not invite the reflexive interaction these objects promised their subjects (toddlers).

Despite some differences, the new design for Park House that is fresh and light with the bright open-plan dining area and places to relax offers a homelike atmosphere, which together with the friendly and caring staff provides a safe home for the mothers and their babies. This is shown through the data from the staff and the clients and yet led to interesting commentary from an interview with two architects, James and Derrick:

> We've built them a lovely environment so they can come and get some respite. Get the ability to emotionally . . . recover . . . and if people re-present . . . because in reality yes, it is a much nicer environment than they're used to, depending on their circumstances. . . . It would be interesting to know if you make a place too nice, I mean what's too nice? But if you make a nice

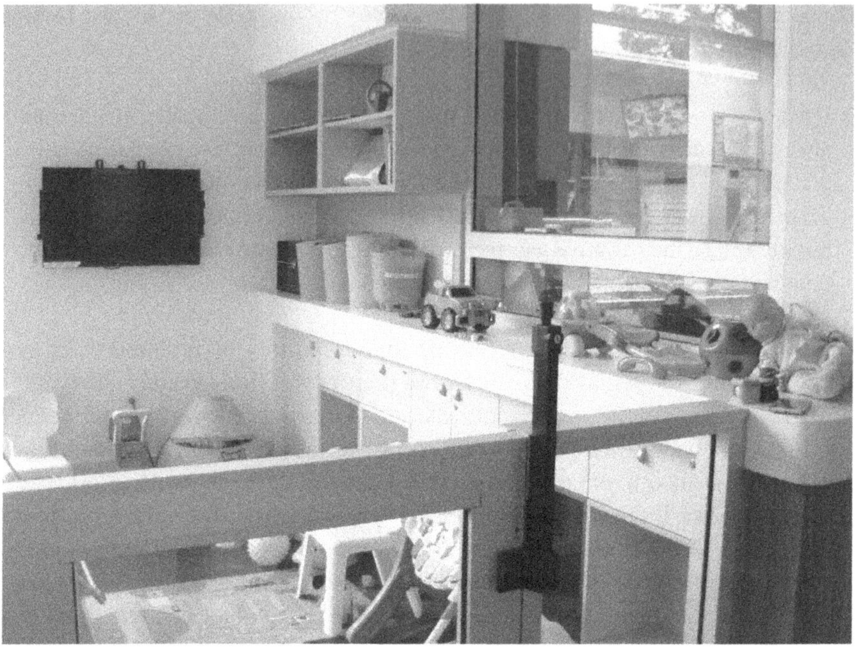

Figure 3.8 Play Pen. *Source*: Photographed by Kathleen Connellan.

> environment, you know, that's relaxing and supporting and enlivening, will people try and get back in, you know, because of that? They come and they have their treatment, they go away back to their own environment and they start to miss being in Park House.

It is a poignant balance: how to create a place with an aura of domesticity that is also a therapeutic space but which is not the mothers "own" home? Domesticity in the ambit of MBU design and occupancy can be misinterpreted. As such, Chryiskou (2014) calls for a new paradigm of domesticity in architecture for mental health. For example, she addresses the concept of "homelike" critically, pointing out that, however, ignoring comfort and choice in the design may compromise therapeutic outcomes. Conversely, and referring to normalization theory, Chrysikou (2014) notes that placing clients in psychiatric units that mimic ordinary housing and homelike-ness can be unrealistic given the diversity of clients. What is alluded to here is that the clients can come from home*less*ness, and therefore the design of an ideal home as sanctuary could even be detrimental.

The interiorities of home can be personalized to equate with interiors of the mind and body (Connellan 2010b, 2018). According to McCarthy (2005, 112), "interiority" in architecture is a concept that shares terms such as "containment, confinement, enclosure, imprisonment, privacy, protection, security, shelter." McCarthy (2005, 112) adds that interiorities are also "immaterial," "mobile," and "promiscuous" to the extent of contamination. There is something of both these seemingly paradoxical interiorities in Redhouse's response to the birth of her child. Redhouse (2019, 11) writes of her sense of catastrophe with the physical reality of having her baby outside instead of inside of her body. Neither her body, her mind, nor her exterior environment was the same after the birth, home in this sense was lost and needed to be found.

Finding home within yourself and for your child when in an MBU may even benefit from extended domestic activities that stimulate and challenge the colliding interiorities of mind, body, and material space. Joseph suggests that there should be:

> working vegetable gardens, a chapel [and] a prayer room, good music rooms that are available 24 hours a day, particularly for bipolar disorder. And they should have art rooms you know where, when you make something out of clay it gets fired, . . . and then it can go to your room or you know they can set up a stall and sell their works or maybe even have a store room where art works are available for patients who are just moving in for a couple of weeks so they can choose how they are going to decorate their own room out of existing stores of art works from patients and ex patients and donations etc. There's a lot that can be done. Unless those ideas are generated by the architects, they're very, very unlikely to ever materialise.

Although Joseph was being interviewed on the unit that is the focus of this study, he brought his specialized research on architecture for mental health to all his responses and comments.

CONCLUDING THOUGHTS

The thematic analysis of the architects' interview data resulted in identifying several themes. They were: evidence; consultation and briefing; the old mortuary; model of care; movement; gardens; safety/privacy; and domesticity.

The most prominent theme by far was the consultation and briefing process. Despite being part of the planning and not a design challenge as such, the issues found in the consultation processes rippled through design, construction, and post occupancy of Park House. Many of the architects were keenly aware of the lack of rigorous evidence which shows what a successful mental health unit design is. Evidence-based design and practice-based evidence are catch words in design but they need to be truly evidence informed, that is from various and comparative studies, which in turn will lead to evidence-generating practice. Evidence-based practice, evidence-informed practice, and evidence-generating practice are all philosophically different. Evidence-based practice usually takes particular types of evidence and integrates it into the plan and build; evidence-informed practice is more continuous and consults research at all possible stages of the project, this involves constant review; and ultimately innovative practice that utilizes evidence conscientiously can in turn provide more evidence for future projects if the evaluations are thoroughly executed.

The principal architects went to the consultations relying on existing exemplars and their own professional experience which stretched across two decades for one of the firms. The state health professionals and clinicians also brought their years of experience to the table for consultation. Individuals in both groups harbored dreams of an ideal place for mothers and babies. The ideal of a home in a village with internal and external gardens, and many of its illusions, was conceptualized into the master plans.

Both groups were intent on providing the best possible unit for the mothers, babies, families, and staff, but experiences and opinions differed, thereby affecting the quality and consensus of the consultations. The groups were also not internally homogenous and, at times, spoke with divided voices. The architects who were predominantly men felt that there were too many voices representing Park House, and the staff, who were predominantly women, felt they were not heard. There was also a lack of representation across both groups, with few women architects and an absence of Indigenous voices at the crucial early stages of the planning. The gender imbalances in the consultations may have unsettled both groups with "passion" and "intensity" construed by some of the male architects as an uncomfortable [female] ingredient that impeded the consultation process. This gender discomfort is reflective of an overwhelmingly male architectural profession. "The idea that women were interlopers in the male [architectural domain] . . . held sway long after the institutional barriers had been breached" at revered organizations like the Royal Institute of British Architects (Walker 2000, 28).

There was also a resistance to the overall plurality of voices with the architects requiring a smoother and arguably more singular approach to the consultations. This was further problematized with the lack of appropriate cultural representation, which was a serious oversight that was not heeded when raised at the crucial consultation phase. When Indigenous knowledge was eventually brought to the table, the decision to use the old mortuary as an entrance was overturned, thereby compromising the benefits of north–south orientation and a united entrance portal design.

The effect of multiple "truths" and memories reverberating through heated consultations resulted in a prescriptive brief, difficulties with the return brief, and masterplans that were not reflective of all the communities involved. Ideals of some were not those of others, resulting in a "heterotopia of crisis" and a spatial and psychological segregation where gender, culture, and professional beliefs collided (Daniels 2000, 197). Clinicians believe in "evidence-based practice" as much as the architects believe in "evidence-based design" but these loaded terms need to be reflexively and inclusively informed. This informing process requires time because differing subjectivities may come from painful experiences that in themselves require healing. As Rose (1998) notes "science" can no longer be seen in the harsh light of conservative positivism because it does not produce knowledge. Instead, it produces restricted views filled with epistemological defects. Thoroughly representative consultations that respect, hear, and listen to every voice is not a simple endeavor, especially with restrictive budgets and timelines. Indeed, it may even be considered an impossible task to undertake such an idealistic approach. It appeared that the consultations for Park House resulted in an acknowledgment of parallel democracies whose separate truths were suspended in the service of expediency (Fry 2011).

Consultations should instead be part of the evidence loop and, as suggested by two of the architects, a substantial component of the budget should be built into gathering and tracking the progress of every stage of the project from its inception to at least five years after occupancy (Connellan et al. 2013; International Living Future Institute 2019). These evaluations should be incorporated into the clinical follow-through with users of MBUs as they transition back into their homes and communities (Connerty et al. 2016; Vliegen et al. 2010, 2013; Wan et al. 2007). The different disciplinary languages for pre and post occupancy evaluations require translation and consensus before consultations can be effective. At present there are architects, interior architects, landscape architects, planners, engineers, health administrators and many different clinicians, each with his/her own professional language (Pearce 2018). Pearce (2018) suggests a "network of methods" rather than a "network of experts" to arrive at clearer understandings of spatial design. However, translating terminology and methods across disciplines is not enough, critiques of gendered subjectivities need to be imbedded into the language. This involves rethinking architectural practice "as text as well as building" (Rendell 2000, 233).

Languages that are transformed into thoughtful practice can be effectively used to translate multiple truths in a way that is acceptable to all. These transformations into inclusive design can be seen as "vectors of force" across the psy disciplines (Rose 1998). One would assume that the garden is surely a place of such inclusion and positive power. However, the gardens of Park House, which were a key focus of the architects, were not equally understood as therapeutically functional spaces by all. One architect claimed gardens are "never properly briefed" and are taken for granted with inadequate integration into the therapeutic milieu. Despite this, and the disappointing impediment of thermal stability taking precedence over fresh air and open garden doors, Park House was designed into the functionality of the gardens. The intention was to treat gardens as an intrinsic part of the interior space. From ethnographic observations and photographs, they appeared bathed in light, carefully landscaped, and equipped with pleasing outdoor furniture, including accessible play equipment. All these elements aimed to invite the mothers into their space and result in the most successful design aspect of Park House along with the surrounding green areas that link all the units on the hospital campus. The architects were proud of them and the occupants appeared to enjoy them. In this way a model of care premised upon the person at the center is mirrored with the garden at the center thus providing a fertile and potentially salutogenic ground for healing (Chrysikou 2014; Golembiewski 2010).

The constant movement through the light filled spaces was a concerted design effort to invigorate a possibly static and "sick" built environment. The flow of human movement parallels mobilities of meaning because, as Massey (1994, 12) notes, "social relations are never still." Bringing life through natural light and free movement which, in turn, generated conversation is one of the most positive effects noted in our observational data. However, ironically, and contrary to most architects' objections to plurality in the consultations, these architects embraced postmodern multiplicity in their flexible open-plan and multipurpose spatial design of Park House. It is an accepted interior design principle that spatial movement and circulation should be designed so that no spaces are simply transitory pathways and that all spaces have interest and distractions designed into them (Edwards 2011). In this way spaces operate as linked pathways and "shifting zones" (Rose 1998). The architects succeed in doing this so the clinical functionality of the spaces is domesticated into a more relaxed flow.

The interior of the MBU offers a kind of repeatable place to practice mothering; its domestic milieu overlaps with its therapeutic milieu. As such, interiors of the mind and interiors of the domestic space require a reciprocal balance. In an MBU both internal and external interiorities are sites of healing. What may seem "normal" home comforts to some clients could appear as luxuries to others and create an imbalance that might impede their recovery in the accommodation that they return to. Chapter 2 of this book pointed out the importance of follow-up after discharge. Therefore, the balance between homeliness and homelike-ness is important for our study on MBUs because after discharge into the community and into the mother's own home, the difference may be extreme.

The idea of only being at home with oneself when the baby remains safely "inside" is a challenge to both psychological and architectural space. The separation at birth, but subsequent reintegration that is required of the mother in her home space, is profound. The terrors of bearing a child and raising it from helpless vulnerability to an independent human being continue to bear down on mothers despite supposed changes in society. Massey (1994, 170) stretches social relations beyond previously established material boundary experiences, including those of the body. It is when feminist appraisals like this become mainstream that there may be less pressure on mothers.

Units like Park House go some way to address the panic encountered with perinatal illnesses. MBUs divert and "redirect" risk of harm to that of the safe "psychological gaze" (Rose 1998, 94). In the ambit of this gaze the mother is encouraged to regain a sense of home and self. This gaze is therefore not the panoptic eye of institutional surveillance; instead, it is domesticated into a home-style atmosphere. The nurses' station is not the watch tower, it is set aside as a stop off point opening out watchfulness into potentially organic clinical interactions. Visibilities and invisibilities merge in a spatial design that has suspended the grid of essentialist order (Rose 1998, 1999). Technologies of surveillance morph beyond the baby monitors to the more human technologies of care. These "techniques of visualisation" (Rose 1998, 108) operate in plain sight and may contribute to a "new democratic legitimacy" in the healing and empowering of unwell mothers (Rose 1998, 88).

More evidence is certainly required, but the departure from reductive and rationalist modernist spaces to one that is a design based more on nature's geometry must surely bring about a change in the symbolic order (Agrest 2000, 360; Massey 1994, 182). The Vitruvian male body (with arms and legs outstretched to provide the classical proportions) remains subliminally present in many public buildings, but the Park House design departs in some way from that essentialism. Nonetheless, the main architects were men; men designing a unit for mothers and babies as well as predominantly female staff. Gender cannot and must not be ignored. Perhaps Rose (1998, 65) is right in saying that the essentialism of a rational [male] modernist order cannot risk the "irrationality" of postmodernism. This type of postmodernism incorporates feminisms which resituate the body in space. Agrest (2000, 359) makes the point that "woman not only has been displaced/replaced at a general social level throughout the history of architecture, but more specifically, at the level of body and architecture." Referring to Renaissance architectural writing, Agrest (2000, 363) reminds us that male architects may substitute their own body's lack to bear a child, to that of giving birth to a building. In this way the architect is both "mother" and "nurse" in the striving to make the building good, strong, beautiful and healthy (Agrest 2000, 363).

This chapter has provided a basis for understanding the design process of Park House, an MBU for mothers, partners, and their babies or toddlers when clinical help is not enough and they need a space to become well and whole. We interrogated how gender is a factor in the design decisions and their outcomes. No finite answers are available but the lived experiences of the users illustrate the complexities of gender across the predominantly male profession of architecture and the overwhelmingly female domain of perinatal nursing and motherhood.

Chapter 4

The Space

Ethnographic Observations

This fourth chapter focuses on the built space within Park House. Specifically, this chapter presents an analysis of our ethnographic observations undertaken within Park House across a two-month period. As outlined in chapter 2, the purpose of the observations was to examine how the space functions, how the space is used, and what effects the space appeared to produce. As such, this chapter explores each of these topics in turn, focusing first on functionality in terms of light, sound, and observation, second on space use in terms of mealtimes and conviviality, and third on the effects of the space in terms of a sense of homeliness within Park House. As we demonstrate, the observed functions, use, and effects of the space in many ways intersect with the intentions of the architects of Park House, as outlined in chapter 3, and the experiences of Park House as elaborated by staff in chapter 5, and service users in chapter 6. Importantly, however, as researchers, our observations offer a critical vantage point on the perspectives of these stakeholders. In other words, while we certainly would not claim that we were entirely neutral parties in the context of the ethnographic observations, we nonetheless undertook observations with a functionalist approach.

This claim about our neutrality (or otherwise) as researchers is an important one to elaborate further. The aim of the ethnographic observations, as outlined above, was to examine, as external parties, how the space within Park House is used, and how such usage potentially produces particular effects. Yet, no matter how quietly we sat, or how unobtrusive we tried to be, our presence was often noted. Some staff asked us, often multiple times, what we were doing in the space. Service users and staff occasionally sought us out to make comments about the space, once they understood our role as researchers. Babies and toddlers smiled at us. And in occupying the space of Park House, even in a liminal way, we too played a role in its operations: by the very fact of observing the space, we drew attention to it *as a constructed space*. In other words, the very fact of observing made visible the fact that Park House is a space built for a specific purpose, and as such it is a space that may or may not fulfill its brief. As such, even when adopting a relatively neutral position (i.e., we did not take up invitations from staff to engage in conversational evaluations of the space during the ethnographic observations phase of the project), our mere presence indicated that there was something to be evaluated.

The analysis presented in this chapter, then, is a situated analysis. It is situated in the sense that we were located within a space to which we were nominally outsiders, but within which we needed to orient ourselves as, to a degree, insiders. In other words, while we came into Park House as outsiders, our interest in and interactions with the space and its users, over time, rendered us to a degree as insiders: we came to know the rhythms of the space, to be seen as "familiar others" within the space, and thus to have a relationship to the space. Our analysis is also situated in that our positionality was not an omnipotent one. We did not simply sit in front of a bank of monitors and observe the space (though such monitors did exist, as we explore below). Rather, we sat in the unit itself. We sat in dining areas, in outdoor areas, in corridors, in staff rooms, in lounge areas, and in the nurses' station of Park House. The observations undertaken in each of these areas are thus situated and partial: at any given moment, our observations were focused on a specific space. This partiality, however, coheres to form an overall "impression" of Park House, one that, in presenting our analysis below, we seek to tease apart to explore some of its constituent parts.

FUNCTIONALITY

At its most basic, and as outlined in chapter 2, the space of Park House functions to house parents (almost exclusively mothers) and their babies, so as to facilitate maternal well-being, and thus to promote positive relationships between mothers and their babies. As we saw in chapter 3, however, this seemingly straightforward goal is far from simple. Housing mothers and their babies is not a neutral exercise. Rather, it requires the production of a space where, it is believed, healing can occur. Contrarily, however, a healing space is not exempt from occupational health and safety requirements that may, at times, run counter to what we know about how healing spaces function. Further, housing, healing, and occupational health and safety may also sit (un)comfortably alongside the aesthetics of architects who seek to design a space that is not simply functional, but is also visually appealing. In this section, then, we focus on how functionality may sit (uncomfortably) alongside purpose and aesthetic appeal.

Light and Sound

Based on our previous experiences undertaking ethnographic observations in an acute mental health ward (Authors 2015), much of our focus in observing the space within Park House was on the function of light and sound. In terms of the former, we were interested in how natural lighting was used within the space of Park House, and how artificial lighting was used to supplement natural light. In terms of the latter, we were interested in how the space itself carried noise: noise from doors opening and closing, shoes on floors, and perhaps most importantly in an MBU, how the sound of voices, and in particular babies crying, carried within the space.

As outlined in chapter 3, the central area of Park House—the dining area—made use of large windows, looking out into two garden areas. This provided for a pleasant outlook for occupants within this central space. At the same time, however, the use of large windows necessitated a highly regulated heating and cooling system that, at times, produced significant discrepancies between internal and external ambient temperatures. In our ethnographic observations we noted that movement between spaces—both from outside to inside and between different spaces within Park House—produced significant changes in temperature. While this cycling of temperatures may, to a degree, replicate shifting temperatures in other built environments such as family homes, in Park House the use of large swathes of glass potentially exacerbated temperature differentials, thus creating the necessity for a more tightly regulated environment than might be the case in other spaces.

Further in terms of light, the large windows located in the dining area were themselves not neutral entities. Windows serve to frame an area, and can be used to create a visual focal point. In the dining area, and as noted above, the windows looked out to two separate garden areas. Figure 4.1 shows the view from the dining area out into a small courtyard area. Figure 4.2 shows the view from the second, larger, outdoor area, looking back through the windows into the dining area. As can be seen in the first image, while the framing of the scene might be considered aesthetically pleasing (given the use of a colored wall, plants, and decorations), it is a scene framed by walls. The light that comes from these windows, then, serves to illuminate the constraints of the space as much as they serve to illuminate the space of the dining room itself. The visual emphasis on the wall outside the window and the relatively constricted nature of the outdoor space framed in the first image serve as a reminder that the space of Park House is a constrained space. Light, in other words, floods everywhere, but occupants of the space, and mothers in particular, are not similarly suffuse: their movement is constrained by walls.

By contrast, the second image allows for a much more open vista. This is a product of the fact that the outdoor area included in this second image is a

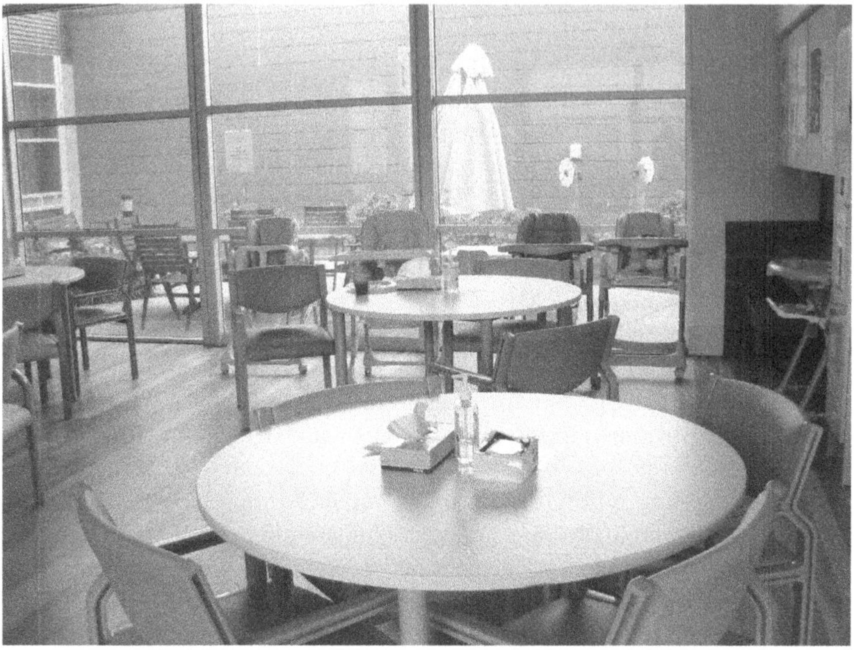

Figure 4.1 Dining Area Looking through to Small Courtyard. *Source*: Photographed by Kathleen Connellan.

much larger space. There is arguably less of a disjuncture between the flooding of light in this garden space, and a sense that movement is restricted. At the same time, however, the sense of restriction is not absent: this outdoor area is again an internal area, bounded on all sides by the internal walls of Park House. Light that comes into this garden, then, is a light contained by walls. This sense of containment is exacerbated by the fact that while this garden area is pleasantly landscaped, over the roofline almost nothing can be seen other than the sky. Nothing can be seen of other buildings, and very little at all can be seen of the trees that form the landscape *outside* of Park House. This garden area, then, even if larger than the smaller courtyard area included in the first image above, it still a bounded area, one that offers more access to light, and which serves to illuminate the dining area, but which nonetheless reiterates the walled nature of Park House.

Moving out from the dining area, by contrast, natural light was much less commonly used. This is understandable, given the need for sleeping spaces to create a climate of restfulness, for both mothers and babies, and to provide privacy in spaces such as staff consulting rooms. Artificial lighting was thus a key feature of spaces such as internal corridors, the nurses' station, bedrooms, nurseries, and consulting rooms. We noted, however, that the lighting

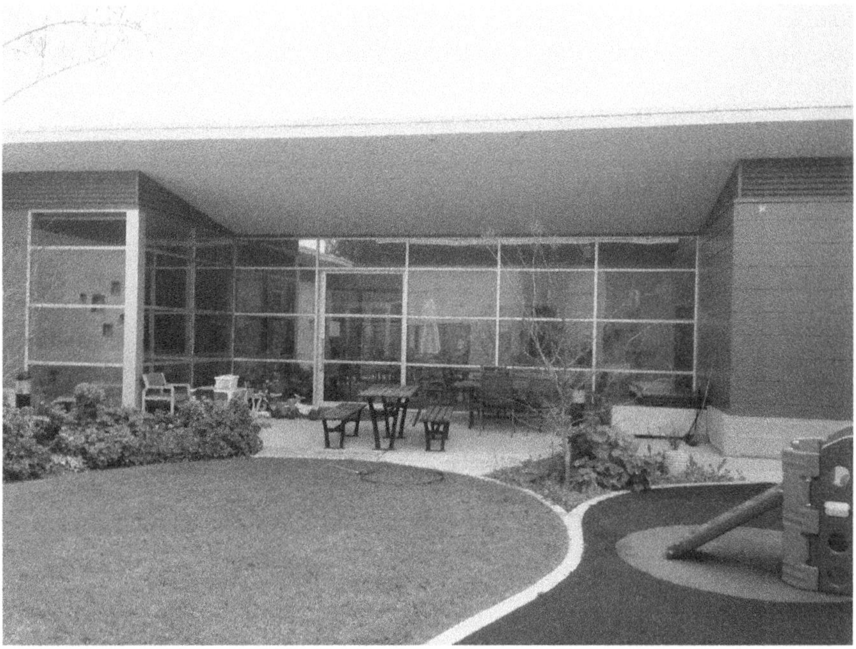

Figure 4.2 Larger Outdoor Area Looking into Dining Room. *Source*: Photographed by Kathleen Connellan.

in these spaces was often inconsistent. In some spaces overhead lighting casts shadows that could make it difficult to read. In some spaces lighting appeared to be on a timer, and was motion activated, yet the activation of such lighting was not always consistent. Also noticeable was a distinction in lighting between the dining room and nearby common areas, the bedroom wing of Park House, and the consulting/staff wing of Park House. Moving between these spaces was akin to moving between distinctly different thematic areas. Common areas were marked by natural lighting, consulting/staff areas were marked by a primacy of artificial lighting, and bedrooms and nurseries marked by often dimmed artificial lighting. While the use of thematic lighting areas might also occur in family homes, in Park House it is served to mark out areas of differing degrees of openness. The consulting/staff area, for example, was a locked area, inaccessible to mothers other than if swiped through by staff. Bedrooms were marked as private areas, though they were accessible to staff in case of emergency. Lighting themes, then, implicitly spoke to these demarcations between accessible, inaccessible, and private spaces.

In a similar way, sound in Park House operated to create thematic zones. Shared areas such as the dining room, formula room, bathrooms, and hallways were all floored in highly resonant materials, namely floating floor boards. This flooring was to an extent aesthetically appealing as well as being functional (i.e., capable of withstanding high traffic as well as spills). In another way, however, it was less than functional. Many of our ethnographic notes comment on the noise of staff shoes "clicking" on the floors, both alerting us to the impending presence of an individual and serving as a form of almost intrusive distraction. By contrast, in the nurses' station, bedrooms, and consulting/staff areas, the floors were carpeted. Here footsteps were muted, adding to the overall thematic feel of these areas as less accessible, or less intended to accommodate a sense of awareness of impending presence.

Further in terms of sound, the use of resonant flooring had implications for the movement of sound. In our observations undertaken when we were located in the communal areas with resonant flooring, we could readily hear sounds travelling from other areas, though somewhat disconcertingly, it was not always easy to discern where the sound was coming from, or even what exactly the sound was. The disconcerting nature of these sounds was of note to us, given the needs of the people housed in Park House, for whom unwanted thoughts or distractions may be exacerbated by the movement of sounds that are hard to interpret.

Conversely, in areas such as the nurseries and bedrooms, the muffling of sounds by carpet meant that it could be harder for mothers to know, for example, if their child was crying, a point we take up in more detail in chapter 6. While the nurseries had monitors so that staff could be aware if a child was crying in one of the nurseries (or if a mother or child was upset in one of the bedrooms), these required active monitoring, which was not always possible. Further, this requirement of monitoring meant that only certain people were positioned as appropriate monitors: mothers did not have portable baby monitors that they could take with them when moving through Park House, so that they could monitor a sleeping baby. Given that, ultimately, the task of Park House is to increase a sense of maternal competency, the apportioning of auditory monitoring primarily to staff potentially did not align with the goal of increased maternal ownership of child monitoring. Certainly, being able to "switch off" from monitoring a child might be important for mothers feeling overwhelmed, but the design of the space did not easily allow for mothers to step back in to monitoring their child, should they desire to do so.

Finally in terms of sound, it was not only the case that in spaces where flooring was highly resonant that sounds appeared to echo and travel. It was also the case that, even in spaces with carpeted floors, noise was an issue. This was especially so in the bedroom wing of Park House. As was the case for all of the doors in the building; the doors in the bedroom wing were heavy, with locking mechanisms that produced a significant noise when doors were shut, especially if those shutting the doors were not careful in their actions. As we mentioned in chapter 3, in our observations we noted that staff commonly let doors slam shut, meaning that sleeping babies could be easily woken up. This was such a concern within Park House that staff had taken to placing small towels along the edges of doors so as to muffle sounds when doors were closed, especially in the bedroom wing. While a functional solution to an evident problem, the use of towels wedged in doors was neither an aesthetically pleasing solution nor was it a solution without problems: in many ways, it potentially reduced privacy for mothers when in their bedrooms. It also potentially reduced a sense of safety, given that other people (including other service users) could enter a bedroom at any time.

Practices of Observation and Surveillance

Again drawing on our experiences in an acute mental health ward (Authors 2012), a focus of our ethnographic observations was on how service users were observed (or not) by staff at Park House. In many ways, as outlined above, the use of natural light via large windows in the dining area was a potentially positive feature of Park House. At the same time, when sitting in this space, we were mindful that the dining area, as both a communal area and as an area that served as a thoroughfare between the bedroom wing and the consulting/staff wing, potentially served an observational purpose. Staff frequently moved through the space, allowing for the informal observation of mothers in the space. This was potentially necessary, given the location of the nurses' station, which did not immediately look over all common areas.

The larger outside area was also an area that, in our observations, produced mixed responses. On the one hand, it was a pleasant area, one that included play equipment for children, space to run around, and benches for mothers, visitors, and staff to sit on. On the other hand, we noted in our observations, and as can be seen in the second image above, that when outside, it was hard to see into the building. This could mean that for mothers in the space, it would be difficult to discern if they were being observed: whether from staff passing through the dining room, or staff sitting in the nurses' station that overlooked the garden. Further adding to the panopticon nature of this garden was its aforementioned boundedness, and the fact that three sets of doors leading to the garden were at times locked, depending on events within Park House and the weather. Indeed, in one of our observational sessions we noted that it was slightly worrying that we could, in effect, be locked in the garden. In many ways, then, the garden offered a simulacrum of an outdoor area, incorporating the standard expected features of a playground, but also encompassing potentially regulatory and observational features.

Finally in terms of observations, when sitting in different areas of Park House, we were mindful of the presence of security cameras. To our eye, these were not always readily evident as such, and certainly were not marked as security cameras. Mothers staying in Park House would likely be aware that they were being monitored, and it was no secret that the nurses' station housed screens that displayed the rooms surveilled by the security cameras. Yet at the same time, the placing of the cameras, the construction of the space as in many ways a homely space (as we will explore below), and the salience (or not) of surveillance, may have meant that mothers were not always aware that they were being observed. Admittedly, mothers give tacit consent to observation upon admission to Park House (and sometimes observations occurred to ensure women's safety), yet this does not mean that consent is not fraught. Indeed, in her own ethnography of an MBU, Masciantonio (2015) notes that mothers were seen as having no capacity as consenting to observation: it was taken as a given. Certainly, the function of Park House is at least in part to observe service users. Yet at the same time, the question we raise here is whether or not the *design* of the space served to incorporate surveillance in ways that were potentially disingenuous, or at least in ways that served to normalize if not to render invisible practices of surveillance. Whether or not staff made use of these design features is another matter, one that we take up in the following chapter.

THE USE OF THE SPACE

In this section we turn to consider how the space was used by staff and service users. Importantly, our observations did not per se include observations of individual people: we did not observe therapy groups or individual sessions with mothers. Our observations of the space, nonetheless, included observations of how people moved within and used the space. In contrast to the previous section, then, where our focus was very much on the built space as itself an entity, functioning with seeming intent upon service users and staff, in this section we focus in turn on how service users and staff used the built space.

Mealtimes

In our reading of the literature on MBUs, we could not identify any research on the meanings and utility of mealtimes. We did, however, identify research on mealtimes in geriatric psychiatric wards. This research (Bryon et al. 2008) suggests that mealtimes can serve an important purpose. Mealtimes can provide routine, they can provide a sense of community, they can provide a sense of competency (in terms of feeding oneself or, in an MBU, also feeding one's child), and they can provide opportunities to create shared traditions and pastimes (such as celebrating key events like birthdays and holidays). As can be the case in any context, then, mealtimes are an important feature of residential psychiatric facilities, and this was very much the case in Park House, though their importance, at least during our observations, was highly regulated by institutional demands.

As noted above, the dining area was a central feature of Park House. It provided a shared gathering area where mothers, their children, their visitors, and staff could come together to share a meal. Meals were served routinely throughout the day, though mothers could also bring in (or have brought in) their own food, which they could prepare in a dedicated "client kitchen." This kitchen, as is evident in figure 4.3, however, while providing mothers with a space in which they could prepare food, was a highly regulated space, one that again created a simulacrum of a domestic kitchen as much as it was a space tightly bound by institutional restrictions.

The kitchen space was bounded by child gates, with a sign clearly stating "no children allowed in kitchen." While the occupational health and safety reasons for this sign are readily discernible, it served to create a nonnormative domestic space, where mothers might be preparing food for themselves or their children, but had to do so separated from their children. Furthermore, as both an institutional space and a shared space, the "client kitchen" was marked by multiple signs instructing service users how to use the space, including in terms of hygiene, safety, and tidying up. Again, it is readily discernible why

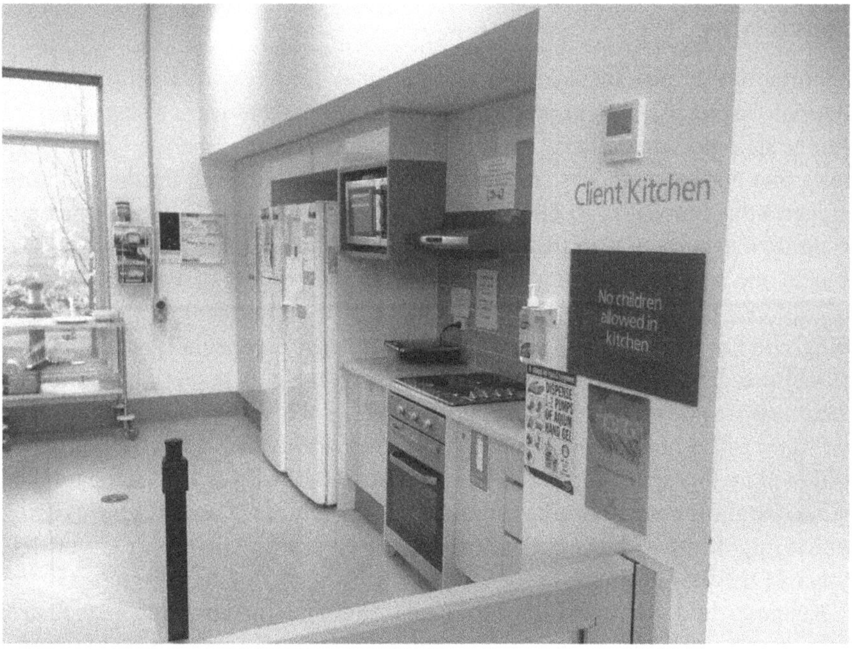

Figure 4.3 Client Kitchen. *Source*: Photographed by Kathleen Connellan.

such instructions were necessary, but they nonetheless served to demarcate the kitchen from a domestic kitchen, instead marking it as an institutional space. In our observational notes, we remarked that it was striking that while the "client kitchen" allowed mothers the relative freedom to prepare their own food, in the fridge food was marked according to the name of the owner. In our reading of the space, this served to reiterate not simply that this was a shared space—as might be common in shared accommodation—but that it was an institutional space, one marked by boundaries and rules.

When observing mealtimes, we noted that the early times at which meals were served (e.g., dinner at 5:00 p.m.) were redolent of hospital mealtimes. On the one hand, then, mealtimes were family-like, yet on the other hand they were regulated by institutional routines. Admittedly, the introduction of clear routines may be good for some mothers, yet at the same time they likely do not reflect meal timings in domestic spaces. The relative oddness of mealtimes was in some ways reflected in how mothers and visitors who joined them during mealtimes made use of the space and time designated for eating. Typically, those eating spent relatively short periods of time in the dining area, often eating fairly quickly and then leaving for another space. Further, not all service users ate at the allocated time, instead saving something for later or opting to prepare their own food.

Conviviality

Importantly, despite the oddness of mealtimes (in terms of timing), and the institutional restrictions upon the "client kitchen," there were times when the dining area did appear to be used to create conviviality. Shaftoe (2012) suggests that convivial spaces are those where people "linger." Further, Shaftoe suggests that convivial spaces are those were the space is legible as one open to particular purposes. In the case of conviviality, then, a space must be legible as one where "lingering" is possible. In the context of Park House, and as explored earlier in this chapter in terms of light and sound, the bedroom wing was not readily legible as a space for lingering, especially when it came to visitors. The two service user lounge areas, while potentially convivial spaces, were somewhat odd spaces, one out of the way and very quiet, and the other often noisy due to a television that was constantly on (though we will explore this space further below in terms of homeliness). This meant that, again, the dining area became the most readily legible space for conviviality, which might in part have been a product of its size: it was much larger than either of the lounge areas.

Kennedy and Fortune (2014), in their research in an acute psychiatric unit, suggest that the women they interviewed wanted more private spaces, including so they could entertain visitors. By contrast, research by Johannson,

Skärsäter, and Danielson (2007) undertaken in a locked psychiatric ward suggested that service users appreciated opportunities to be together, including in shared spaces with visitors. Similarly, in our observations in Park House, shared spaces were where visitors were commonly entertained, primarily in the dining area but also, weather permitting, the outdoor areas. During one mealtime observation we witnessed a staff member offering a partner to join in the meal, noting that "he was part of the family." This invitation to conviviality is important, as it potentially signaled that what might otherwise be seen as a clinical space to visitors was legible as a space to "linger."

At other times we noted a sense of "friendliness" when visitors were present, with multiple mothers and their visitors sharing the dining space, with people looking at and remarking on one another's children. This sense of conviviality was at times extended by mothers and their visitors to staff, who were referred to using kinship referents (e.g., referring to a female staff member as "aunty"), again in shared spaces. Often it was visitors who initiated these types of interactions and affinities, potentially signaling that the role of the space was seen as a convivial one, a role that may have served to normalize the institutional nature of the space.

Conviviality, then, may not simply be a product of a space, as Shaftoe (2012) suggests. It may also be produced *despite* the space. In other words, in Park House, marked in many ways as an institutional space, and one not necessarily predisposed to conviviality, some service users found ways to mark the space as convivial: by small gestures or occupancy of the space that allowed for a sense of wanting to "linger." As we explore in the following section, certainly aspects of the built space appeared to help facilitate a sense of homeliness. Importantly, however, a semblance or simulacrum of homeliness does not necessarily translate into an experience of homeliness. Nonetheless, in this section we have suggested that, at least for some service users, they found ways to create conviviality, either by using or reframing the space as one in which they could linger and feel at home.

EFFECTS OF THE SPACE

As we alluded to above, there was a sense in which the built space of Park House was intended to evoke a sense of being at home. Certainly as we noted in chapter 3, the architects saw this as part of their remit: to create a homely space. Yet as the title of this book would suggest, spaces such as Park House are both home and away: they may appear homely or homelike, and may in some ways replicate home life, but they are resolutely institutional spaces. They are ruled by regulations, and designed to serve a purpose that is typically not homely. In an essential, and perhaps necessary way, then, Park

House was always going to be a simulacrum of a home, and it was potentially necessary that the simulated aspects of the built space were readily discernible: it should not be so much like home that service users forget why they were there. With this point in mind, in this section of the chapter we explore how the built space of Park House both evoked a sense of home, but did so in many ways that were readily discernible as not actually being home.

Homeliness

In his exploration of architectural design for psychiatric care, Golembiewski (2010) suggests that such built environments should "mimic" homely spaces. This word "mimic" is important: it reiterates our suggestion above that built spaces such as Park House are meant to approximate, but not entirely replicate, homely spaces, a point we have already introduced in chapter 3, and will take up again in chapters 6 and 7. Research on mental health inpatient units too suggests that such units should be "homelike," but not necessarily a home (Wood et al. 2013). This creates something of a tension, then, in that psychiatric units, including Park House, must manage a fine line between engendering a sense of home, while not seeming too much like home. As the examples below would suggest, it was potentially the case that Park House managed this fine line by including some features that were markers of home, while potentially not including all of the features (or only including certain versions of features) that would make the space truly home.

As suggested earlier in this chapter, televisions were one aspect of Park House that potentially functioned to create a homelike space. In our observations we noted that in one of the service user lounge areas, there was a television always on, even if no one was in the room. Further we noted that the television often screened programs that were not particularly suitable for small children. We wondered if the constant presence of a television served to replicate home spaces where, at least in some households, a television might always be on. This, however, might be a particularly classed iteration of homeliness. Skeggs and Wood (2011), for example, suggest that the constant presence of a television set reflects particular classed values about what watching television means, especially for children. Whether or not this was purposively the case in Park House is beyond the scope of our ethnographic observations, however it does raise the question as to what architects and staff might think constitutes home for service users, and how this reflects particular classed assumptions about service users, a point we explore more in chapter 7.

Returning to the topic of the larger outdoor garden, it was only after several sessions of observation that we noticed a clothesline which was screened behind wooden fencing. As can be seen in figure 4.4, while the screening

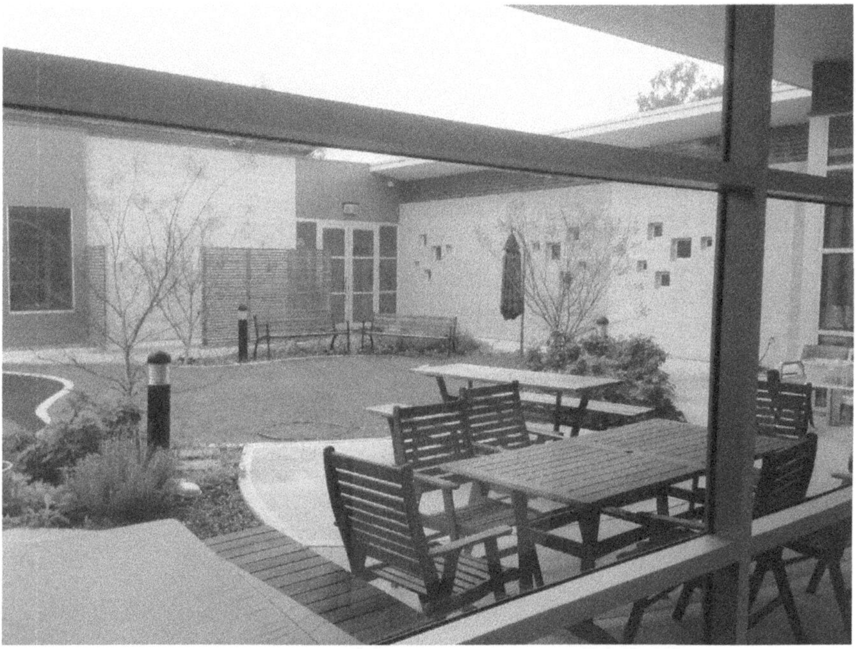

Figure 4.4 View of Large Outdoor Area from Dining Room Windows. *Source*: Photographed by Kathleen Connellan.

served an aesthetic function, it didn't entirely mask the presence of the clothesline. As a domestic space, the existence of a clothesline was important, allowing mothers to wash and dry their clothes. We might suggest that this is more than just a homelike feature of Park House, instead suggesting that a clothesline is clearly redolent of home. Yet situated within the broader confines of the garden space, which as we have argued above was a space regulated by boundaries and reminders about them, the clothesline is both a reminder of home and a reminder that one is away from home.

What also stood out to us in regard to homeliness (or a lack of it), and in contrast to the examples provided above, was a lack of paintings or prints on the walls of Park House in the communal areas. Certainly, as we noted with regard to the "client kitchen," there were many signs instructing service users how to appropriately interact with the space, but there was little by way of decorations. Certainly, not every home will have paintings or prints on the walls, but our previous observations in an acute mental health ward noted the presence of art on the walls and its effects (Authors 2011).

It stood out to us, then, that the communal areas of Park House were largely absent of any kind of decoration. An exception (figure 4.5) was a set of collages created by mothers staying in Park House during art therapy sessions.

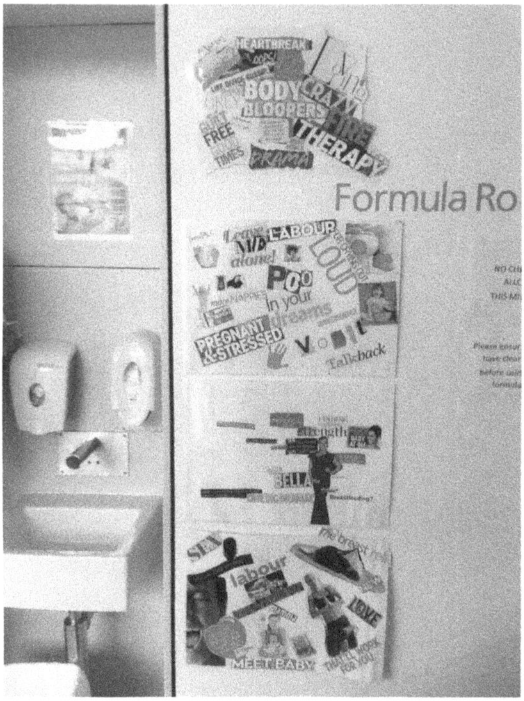

Figure 4.5 Collages Made by Mothers Staying in Park House. *Source*: Photographed by Kathleen Connellan.

The women had cut out words and images from magazines that they felt in some way captured their experiences. As can be seen in the image, this was a powerful and evocative piece of art. Importantly, however, as the image demonstrates, this collage was located on the door of the formula room: it was not on a main wall within Park House, instead located relatively out of the way on the door of a room that is less likely to be seen by visitors. There might well have been a reason for this: aspects of the collage could be seen as challenging. It was in a location that mothers would be likely to see on a regular basis (i.e., when preparing bottles for their children), but as the image suggests, it is a particularly clinical location, redolent with signs about hygiene and safety, and thus not a particularly homely space. Certainly we cannot be specific about the reasons for placing the collage on the door to the formula room, however as is the focus of this section, we can speak to its potential effects: it is relatively out of the way, in a space primarily used by mothers, and it is on the entrance to a space that is also marked by clinical information. As such, although the displaying of the collage potentially honored the women who created it as the product of art therapy, it also situated their work at the clinical margins of Park House, rather than in the communal, convivial spaces, such as the dining area.

An exception to the lack of art in Park House was a print located in the staff/consulting wing. While a pleasant image that suited the space, it was notable to us that it was located in an area to which service users only had restricted access. It is possible that the print was hung by staff of Park House, looking to add some detail to the area of Park House in which they spent a considerable amount of their time. However if this supposition is the case, it raises the question as to why the other, communal spaces of Park House were not similarly decorated, given service users spent so much of their time in the communal spaces. The lack of art in the communal spaces, then, potentially served as a reminder that while aspects of Park House were homelike, it is, at the end of the day, not a home. Indeed, we noted in our observations that the communal spaces of Park House very much felt like a combination of a hotel and a doctor's waiting room, yet such spaces would normally include some sort of decorative features. It was thus all the more noticeable to us that the absence of enhancing features in the communal spaces of Park House spoke, whether intentionally or unintentionally, to the sense of being "home and away" that the built space appeared to evoke.

CONCLUDING THOUGHTS

Following on from chapter 3, in this chapter we have focused thematically on key topics evident in our ethnographic observational notes. Given our interests, it was not surprising that aspects of functionality were central to our observations. Arguably less expected, however, were our observations about mealtimes, conviviality, and homeliness. Certainly these are topics that intuitively "fit" with a focus on built spaces such as Park House, which by necessity combine aspects of home and aspects of the institution. Yet given the relative scarcity of previous research focusing on these aspects of psychiatric spaces (and nothing within the context of MBUs), it is notable to us that to a certain degree these features and effects of the built space were evident within our ethnographic notes, despite a primary focus on the functionality of the space.

Reflecting on the findings presented in this chapter, it is also important to revisit the topic of our role as researchers within the space of Park House. In this chapter we have been, to a certain degree, critical of the design of the space, including the aspects of the space that may present a veneer of homeliness (and thus mask the observational aspects of the space, including the presence of security cameras), and conversely, the aspects of the space that fail in the remit to be homely (i.e., the lack of art). It thus behooves us to be similarly critical of the fact that our presence potentially served as an additional observational layer to the experience of service users. As we noted in the introduction to this chapter, our presence served as a reminder that Park House is a built space that can be evaluated. Yet, our presence may also have served as a reminder that Park House is primarily a space for observations *in general*. Certainly, nearly all service users consented to our observations, but this did not mean that those who consented did not feel compounding forms of observation as a result of our presence. This is a topic that we will take up in the final chapter of this book in greater detail.

It is also of note that in this chapter we made interpretations on the basis of our ethnographic observations, imputing potential meaning (or the lack thereof) of objects within Park House, the potential intentions of architects and staff in Park House, and the potential effects of the built space. Importantly, then, these are our observations, and it is us as researchers and authors who have imputed this meaning. Certainly in some ways the meanings we impute in this chapter align with the views expressed in other chapters in this book by architects, staff, and mothers. But the meanings we attribute are nonetheless those of outsiders. As much as we suggested in the introduction to this chapter that, over time, we become familiar with and comfortable in the space, among our diversity of experiences of children and mental health, we have not spent time housed in a space such as Park House. As a result, while we became familiar with and somewhat comfortable in the space, we were never truly insiders. Rather, we were "known others," sharing something of the experience of the space, but from a very specific subject position (i.e., researchers). Certainly our own experiences of children and mental health, in varying ways, overlay our subject position as researchers, but at no point do they overlap in entirety with the experiences of the service users or staff of Park House.

In many ways our ethnographic observations suggest that Park House to a fair extent fulfilled its brief: it was homelike in some ways, but not so homely as to become a space that mothers would not want to leave. The built space allowed for observations of service users by staff, without these observations being unnecessarily intrusive. It allowed for conviviality and a degree of privacy for service users, without ignoring occupational health and safety requirements. Notably, however, there were aspects of the functionality of the built space that potentially fell short. The effects of noises, particularly with regard to floors and doors, could potentially have negative effects on service users, suggesting that these aspects of the design could be improved. Certainly, as we noted, staff and mothers were finding creative ways (such as wedging bedroom doors with small towels) to address problems related to sound, but these solutions were not ideal, nor particularly aesthetically pleasing or conducive to privacy for service users. This suggests that the findings included in this chapter highlight both strengths and room for growth in terms of the design of purpose built spaces that aim to facilitate well-being.

This would suggest, then, that while it is important that staff are consulted in the process of designing spaces such as Park House (which was the case for the staff of Park House, as we explore in chapter 5), it is also important that service users are consulted. Accompanying such consultations should be evaluations of the space post occupancy, so as to ascertain if the design brief has been achieved. Finally, it is important that spaces such as Park House hold open the capacity for change. Certainly, some fixtures and features are static, and not open to change. Other features, however, may hold the potential for change, including change based on post occupancy evaluations. In the context of Park House, some post occupancy changes were made, though these are primarily related to safety features of the space that were not functioning correctly (e.g., fire sprinklers). Other features required ongoing maintenance, necessitating ongoing evaluations of the space (e.g., on one day of observations we noted that the security monitors in the nurses' station were not working). But beyond this, it is important that changeable features, such as furniture and décor, are seen as features open to change, so as to ensure that the potentially shifting needs of service users can be met. Built spaces such as Park House, then, need to be both static and dynamic spaces, capable of adapting over time. This requirement for adaptation is thus a necessary design feature that may be usefully and purposively incorporated into future purpose builds in the context of design for well-being.

Chapter 5

The Workspace

Staff Perspectives

Much of the literature concerning MBUs has focused on staff perspectives, although this tends to be concerned with staff perspectives of service users and their mental health rather than the space and design of MBUs themselves. However, staff perspectives of the design of MBUs are important in order to understand how the space functions as a workspace as well as a therapeutic one, including how the space may function (or not function) to promote relationships between parents and children and between service users and staff. Moreover, and as noted by Novotná, Urbanoski, and Rush (2011), staff perspectives on, and experiences of, the space in mental health units are also important because they are inextricably linked to the experiences of service users and the quality of the care provided. Previous research has found that staff identify adequate space for private work tasks (e.g., phone calls, report writing), well-designed therapeutic spaces, and safety—including suicide prevention—to all be particularly important considerations in the design of MBUs (e.g., Shepley et al. 2017), which broadly mirrors that of psychiatric units and healthcare settings more broadly (Ulrich et al. 2008). This chapter builds on this research to identify key issues identified by staff in relation to the space within Park House.

The chapter is informed by interviews conducted with fifteen staff, all of whom were women. Staff all held clinical positions, and included nurses, psychiatrists, and psychologists, some of whom also held positions of authority (e.g., unit manager). Many of the staff had worked in the previous MBU, and as such they could compare their experiences of Park House with that of their previous workplace, which led to interesting reflections on space and design. Staff were interviewed in person or over the phone, with in person interviews typically taking place in a private office (although this also often involved walking through the building to show the researchers aspects of the space that they were referring to). Staff were asked a small number of open-ended questions surrounding what was "good" or "bad" in the design of the space, and prompted to consider both their own experiences and those of service users, although, as discussed throughout the chapter, staff typically focused on how the space functioned in relation to the well-being of mothers and their babies or children.

Eight overarching themes were identified through analysis—Issues in the Workspace: Staff Experiences; Privacy versus Clinical Needs; The Therapeutic Space: Accommodating Therapy; Creating Home in an Institution; Smoking; Noise; Accommodating Children in a Mother-Baby Unit; and Flexible Outdoor Spaces Facilitate Parent-Child Relationships. These themes we identified not only because they were the most commonly spoken of by staff but also, following Braun and Clarke's (2006, 2013) approach, because they were the most salient in relation to space and in terms of the position of staff within that space. It is noteworthy in relation to these themes that the staff we spoke to were all women, and that the clients they worked with were also almost always all women.

ISSUES WITH THE WORKSPACE: STAFF EXPERIENCES

As noted above, staff typically oriented to concerns about service users' experiences of the space rather than their own in interviews. However, some did discuss elements of the space which affected them, their experience of their workplace (the MBU), and their interactions with clients and their families. A key example of this was that of the location and design of the nurses' station, which many staff felt was not well designed in terms of privacy and overcrowding due to the demands of an MBU—such as prams and equipment.

In relation to privacy, staff noted that if the door to the nurses' station was open people could enter without someone in another part of the station knowing, leading to the potential for private discussions or telephone conversations to be overheard (see figure 5.1). As Diana noted:

> Someone walks out of the room but leaves the door open and you might be on the phone, you can't see around that corner and then when you get up and you walk around or someone knocks on the door and you realise someone's standing there, so they knock on the open door, you're having a very private conversation on the phone to another agency and this person might have heard it. And then you think, "my goodness, what did they hear?," particularly if it's about that patient, you know, that bit of angst about, what happened then. So I just find the design of the nursing station very difficult.

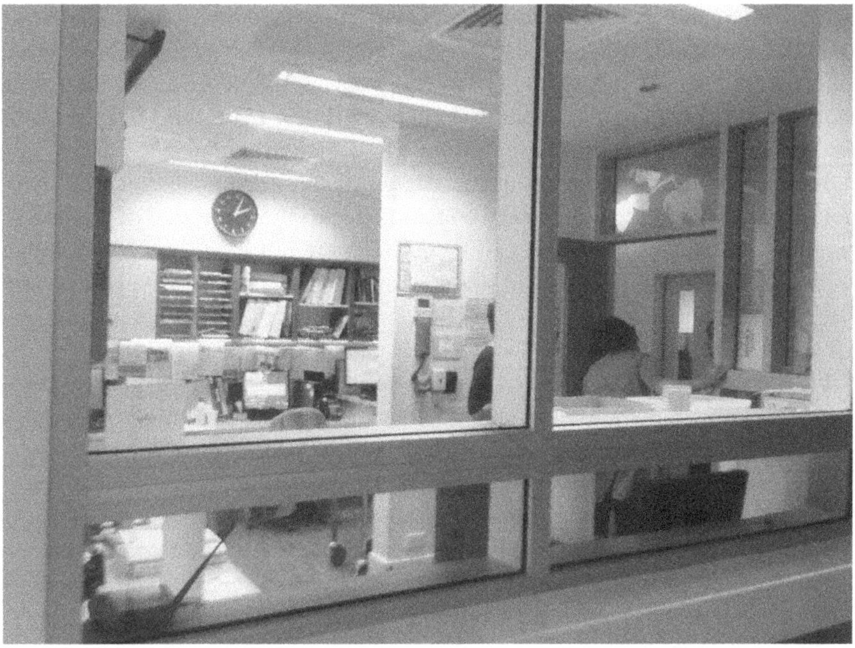

Figure 5.1 Conversation at Nurses' Station Door. *Source*: Photographed by Kathleen Connellan.

Josie also discussed issues relevant to the nurse's station, including the compact space when there were prams or strollers (pushers) present, the noise when there were multiple people talking, and the issue of privacy noted by Diana above:

> The nurses' station. If anyone was thinking through—like, today I was kneeling typing. You can't actually fit anymore chairs than there is in there. And if you've got pushers and . . . . It's pretty tight for space and it's pretty loud and it's hard to hear and whilst it may be soundproof there's an awful lot of sound going on in there . . . often handovers happen in there and they need to be confidential but people are coming in all the time. And you can't necessarily see the door if you're in the back section . . . so if you're having a conversation there or you're on the phone—you picked up the phone and it's [child protection department] saying, "what's the child protection concerns for this family?" and then the mum comes to the door and wants her medication and someone's got the door open—it's like, I can't say a thing. And you don't really want to say, I'm sorry I can't talk now, the person I'm talking about is standing at the door. So it's often really awkward.

Nurses' stations have been the subject of a small amount of previous literature concerning psychiatric units generally, often with a focus on security, surveillance, and their regulatory function (Andes and Shattell 2006). While staff did not specifically discuss observation of service users in these interviews, concerns about privacy were prevalent as seen above, together with practical concerns such as space. As such, staff discussed the MBU in terms of their own experiences and regarding MBU's control of service users.

In addition to concerns about the design of the nurses' station, staff also noted that there were some safety concerns due to the large size of the MBU, meaning that noises in one area of the MBU were not heard easily in another area. Farida told the interviewer about a situation which she felt arose in part due to this issue of design:

> I was struggling one night with a woman who was detained and had managed to pinch a knife from the kitchen and was trying to cut her throat. And I'm pressing my buzzer but the other nurse, because we had toddlers in, thought it was a false alarm. And even though I was yelling out from where I was, nobody could hear me. So it can be problematic, just distance and the degree of soundproofing. Luckily those sort of things happen fairly rarely but it was an interesting situation for a few minutes. I just kept pressing the buzzer and eventually somebody from one of the other wards did come in. But because [of] distance and not being able to hear somebody else it can put spouse members at risk.

In this situation, the large size of the MBU—which was elsewhere discussed as a positive element as seen later in this chapter—created challenges for staff, including in relation to their safety and that of service users.

Another design issue staff noted related to light. While staff generally agreed that the unit was light and airy and that this was positive, they noted that the building was facing the wrong way and "so the blinding sun in the morning and then the afternoon impacts on clients. You can't even see people down the corridor" (Brie). Diana also discussed this, saying:

> Generally the open feel to it and the light coming in is lovely, however, I was a little bit surprised at having the big windows in the main area of the unit facing east and west. So in the morning you get this horrible sun coming in and in the afternoon you get the horrible very hot sun in the summer. And it is just so glary and hard to work in that space.

These observations about light mirror our own as discussed in chapter 4, suggesting that the design of the unit could have considered light—which has been previously identified as important in MBUs by ourselves and others—more carefully (Authors 2015; Ulrich 2008). It also reflects back on the issues we discussed in chapter 3 where there were late changes to the design due to issues with using the Old Mortuary façade as an entrance. In general, however, staff were positive about the overall design of the unit in relation to the way it functioned as a work space.

PRIVACY VERSUS CLINICAL NEEDS

Overall, staff felt that the MBU took into account the needs that mothers may have in terms of privacy, with privacy a frequent topic within interviews. For example, in response to a question about the design of the MBU and its relationship to mental health for clients, Alannah said: "I think generally it will impact positively in that the people have their own room and have their own bathroom. Particularly women, so their own privacy."

Staff noted that bedrooms were generally spacious, and included double beds so that partners and other children could stay overnight, which also met the privacy needs that a family may have. However, some staff noted that the bedrooms for more acute service users were less spacious, and that perhaps this could have been more balanced in the planning stage to ensure that acute service users' needs in this regard were also met. Private bedrooms have previously been identified as supportive of recovery for clients (e.g., Novotná, Urbanoski, and Rush 2011), and so this aspect of the space appears to be important for both therapeutic and autonomy reasons.

Staff also felt that service users were attuned to the potential privacy needs of others, which was important within a shared space. For example, Alannah noted that while the space was small and often crowded, when lots of family were visiting other service users tended to "naturally give each other space." Alannah elaborates: "If someone's outside with visitors, you know, with their kids or something, I do think a lot of times people go 'Oh they're out there. We'll give them that,' you know, patience as well." However, while privacy was identified as a key consideration in the design of the MBU—and one which was likely to affect mental health for service users—there were tensions present in discussions around this topic. In particular, staff noted that while privacy may help to promote mental health, it was also problematic for the specific group of service users within the MBU and their clinical or well-being needs. For example, Alannah also said, "there's some women who aren't that comfortable with other people, and they do tend to go up and isolate themselves in their rooms a bit. And sometimes that's okay—it just depends on what their issues that have brought them here. And, you know, if you're depressed and you're isolating yourself, that's not so good."

Overall, then, staff were positive about the ways in which the MBU afforded privacy to clients and oriented to this in interviews as a key example of a positive element of the space and its design. However, there were tensions in the ability for a space to offer privacy and the need for clients to use the space in ways which met their needs but were also positive for their own mental health—that is, the space is ultimately a therapeutic one and staff felt that it needed to function in such a way that it promoted positive mental health outcomes. Privacy (or at least, only using the space to gain privacy) was seen by some staff as potentially counterproductive to this goal, at least some of the time.

THE THERAPEUTIC SPACE: ACCOMMODATING THERAPY

As noted in the previous theme, staff frequently responded to questions about design by discussing the space with respect to the therapeutic needs of the service users—perhaps unsurprisingly given their roles as clinicians. In particular, staff discussed this aspect of the design in terms of their relationships with service users and the need to build trust and rapport in order to promote well-being. For example, staff frequently highlighted that the design of the MBU meant they were often walking through communal spaces, and in doing so were frequently interacting with service users, building relationships in a casual way (or at least, a way that could be perceived as casual by service users). For example, Alannah said:

> I think it's good because when you go out of our office you go straight into the common area [dining area], so you walk through where people are generally, and you chat . . . and the children chat and talk to you. And so I think that's worked out really well. So you are really quite frequently with them. . . . And it's also sometimes you're waiting to see someone, because they're asleep, the baby's asleep, you know, they're seeing someone else, or you want to do a group or something and so you're kind of just needing to check where things are at. It's not like a set "We're doing this at this time." Sometimes it's, you know, it has to be quite flexible. So you go in, you can just drift in and out and see where things are really quite easily.

This ability to walk through the MBU unobtrusively and observe service users and their babies or children was seen not only as positive in relation to facilitating relationships but also in relation to observing service users and their interactions with their babies. In other words, it also facilitated the purpose of the MBU itself in promoting positive attachment between mothers and their children. As Brie, said: "I'm continuously walking backwards and forwards so I have little snapshots of ability to sort of interact."

However, some staff noted that it could also be problematic that they had to walk through areas where service users regularly spent time, especially if they were rushed and could not stop to talk. Joan highlighted this by outlining a potential scenario:

> And someone was talking about how one of the babies was doing and how the registrar had walked through and said hello to all these other babies. And there was one that was a bit hidden and she didn't see her and the baby apparently and was sort of was like, "hey, you didn't say hello to me." And I am conscious when I walk through like that so given that to get from my office to the nurses' station I've got to go through—I guess I could—really I have to go through without going outside—have to go through a patient communal area which mostly is fine. But there's that thing if I'm really rushed or whatever sort of thing it's like, yes, I say hello to the patients every time and also an awareness of saying hello to everybody. There is issues here sometimes and it depends on particularly with people if we've got a group of people admitted with more vulnerable or tricky personality structures I guess then if I say hello to one patient but not the other they might feel somehow rejected or something like that.

In this regard staff noted challenges when the space functioned both as a practical means of getting from one location to another and as a therapeutic space in which to build relationships with others. In particular, there were difficulties when one use of the space (walking from A to B) outweighed the other (interacting and building relationships) without service users being aware of this distinction. Previous research has similarly highlighted issues with communal spaces and layouts which lead to increased contact between staff and service users, with Novotná and colleagues (2011) noting that this could be problematic not only for staff but also for service users, who do not necessarily want to be around staff all day.

Another issue discussed by some staff in terms of the layout of the MBU was the location of some interview rooms. Constance indicated that these were far away and required unlocking and locking some internal doors on the way, which she felt negatively affected her ability to build trust and rapport with service users by reinforcing the unequal power relationship between them:

> the main interview room that we use is between two locked doors. So you have to walk down the corridor, unlock the first door, down another corridor and unlock the second door before you get into the interview room. Which, look, most of the time doesn't have an impact, but sometimes I'm aware that that adds this kind of sense of foreboding and formality to an interview. So "Let's go and have a talk," and it's kind of you're developing what seems to be a relatively warm rapport, but then to have a discussion about anything you have to unlock two doors, which is sort of somehow symbolic of institution to me.

Here, Constance highlights an issue noted by many staff in the space's ability to accommodate the therapeutic needs of clients—that of frictions between the space as a home and the space as a medical facility or institution. This is discussed further in a later theme, but underlines here the way in which the needs of the institution with respect to safety and security might also be counter to the needs of the institution with respect to building a therapeutic space.

Finally, in relation to the space as therapeutic, staff discussed not only the need to build trust and rapport with service users, but also the need to teach them skills—particularly parenting skills in relation to learning to care for their baby, toddler, or older children. For example, Alannah said:

> For a number of . . . I mean some people come from the country so their partners when they visit need somewhere to stay, unless there's an issue where the partner shouldn't stay, in terms of there might be violence, or that the woman herself needs to learn to do things on their own without, you know, just have some time with their baby on their own. And also they'll sometimes bring in an older child with them, so the mum builds up her skills in caring for a baby and a child. So it is really important there's that space [in the bedrooms]. And even for women in [city name], some of them are really scared to come in, but they are more willing to do so if their partners are here to feel more comfortable. But also the reality is when they go home their partners are going to be there. So the partner gets the opportunity to learn from staff too how to care for their child and how to support the mother.

Here, Alannah indicates that the space needs to at least approximate "home" in some respects, since it is to home that the service users will return when they leave the MBU. Alannah discussed this specifically in terms of bedrooms and the ability for partners to stay the night, again underscoring the positive nature of the unit's large bedrooms.

Overall, staff felt that the space offered some avenues to support the therapeutic needs of service users, but there were several tensions present in terms of the competing demands placed upon the space and its design. These tensions are the focus of the following theme.

CREATING HOME IN AN INSTITUTION

In general, staff participants indicated that the MBU was welcoming and inviting—a space they felt that service users would like to come to. As Alannah said: "I think that people would be happy to come in here." Brie similarly discusses the homely space:

> I think clients are pleasantly surprised that it is fairly peaceful apart from occasionally it's chaotic and all that. But the actual environment here is actually a lot nicer than they might have perceived. Certainly their room, they've got their own bracelet they can get into their rooms, it's a sense of safety. It is a family unit. We talk about safety all of the time and getting well and all those sorts of things. And largely those people who struggle to want to ever come in here we actually struggle to discharge them. We've got people who would like to live here very much so. So that's certainly a common thing that they actually want to stay. And that's, I guess, a supporting environment as well.

In addition to being therapeutic, staff in a research project by Novotná and colleagues (2011) noted that an "attractive" design reduced the stigma of coming to a mental health unit. Stigma was not specifically discussed by staff in this project, however this was implied—for example, Brie indicated that the space was so successful in achieving a sense of home that the MBU sometimes "struggle[d] to discharge" service users. Joan agreed with this, saying that the space was "more homely and less 'hospitally' than expected" and that service users and their families were often "surprised, they thought that it doesn't feel like a hospital that it's more homelike." In particular, Joan noted small design features of the MBU which they felt made it home—for example, small handprints in the outpatient's lobby (see figure 5.2): "These are really small things but one of my favourite things at the ward is in the—if you come in from the outpatient side where there's that little orange bench and kitchen area—in the glass we look at through to the small courtyard it's frosted glass and there's child hand prints in there."

Joan went on to note that creating a homely space was particularly important for other children coming to visit their mothers and siblings:

> I think the fact for any kids who are anything from pre-schoolers up can be a bit—mum's had a baby and sometime in the last, maybe quite recently have disappeared and come home and disappeared again—are not really sure what's going on and stuff it can be a bit hard. And I think it's good that the environment is less 'hospitally' as such. I wouldn't say it seems quite homely but it's not as scary as some other hospital would be which probably makes it a bit easier for some of the kids coming to visit.

Interestingly, some of the design features of the space which were noted as creating a sense of home also doubled as necessary within an institutional environment—such that there was not always conflict between these two roles for the space. An example of this were the en suites in the bedrooms. These were discussed by staff as creating privacy for service users and facilitating a sense of home where people could use their own bathroom. However,

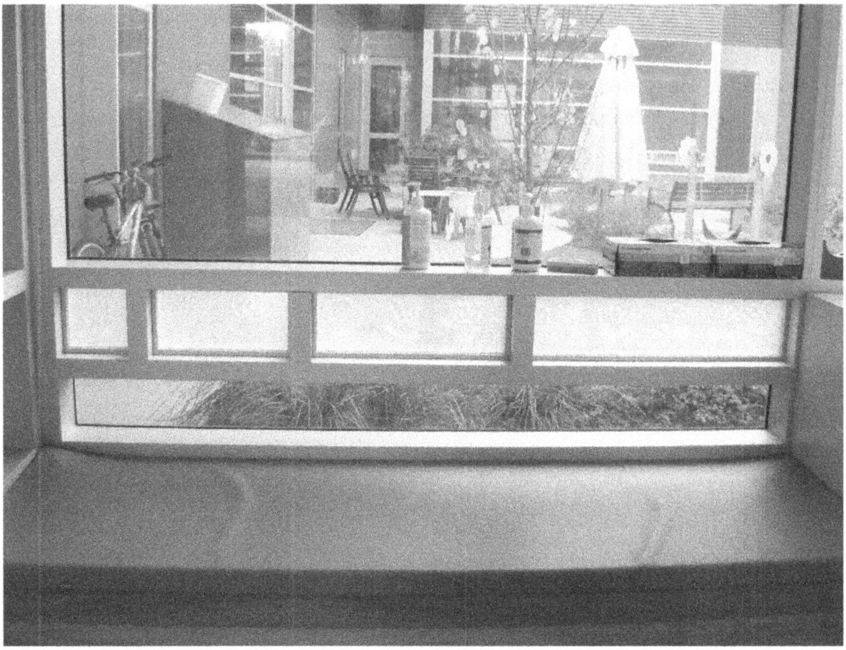

Figure 5.2 Glass Handprints, Window Seat in Outpatients' Lobby. *Source*: Photographed by Kathleen Connellan.

separate en suites also functioned as infection control, where Mathilde, for example, noted that having en suites "makes it easier" to control the spread of infections such as gastro, because "we're pretty strict otherwise with sending people off [home]."

However, other staff noted a range of elements of the space which made creating "home" in an institution difficult, leading to some strain in the perception of the MBU as homely. Chief among these was the fact that ultimately the space is a communal one and has to be shared with other people who are unknown to each other, including the staff who looked after both service users and their babies. As Constance said: "The shared nursery spaces are, like some patients felt to be a bit strange, they don't like having their babies in with somebody else . . . and it's also just, I guess, a bit different to what they might be doing at home. And sometimes they do complain that sort of living in a communal space can be quite challenging."

Staff also highlighted other elements of the space which created tensions with the sense of home, particularly those which were necessary within a functioning institutional space. An example of this was the centrally controlled air conditioning within the building. Joan noted:

> Air conditioning is in—some rooms are freezing—this is on the cooler side but not as cold as my office—some are too hot. And I think when you've got little babies and the mums are saying the rooms are freezing and they can't sleep and sleep is really important for mums who need to be getting better—and all we can do is get an extra blanket, so some of those things.

Another example of this was the presence of microphones in bedrooms, with some staff indicating that while they were necessary for safety, they disrupted the homely feel of the bedrooms—and indeed that the sense of privacy in bedrooms was ultimately an illusion. Diana said:

> The idea is to say to them that if there's some reason you want to have the microphone turned off—because we can turn it off and on in the nursing station—but keeping in mind that usually when they're admitted they're very unwell. And people who are unwell, whether it's physical or mental health issues, struggle to process new information so really you'd have to say that on a daily basis which actually probably is the thing. Yeah that [privacy] is a delicate balance especially when we've got all the bedrooms . . . We do on admission we do tell the clients that there is intercoms in all the rooms and that's basically for the babies crying and for safety. We can have it a certain volume so if somebody's yelling or shouting in the room or looks stressed we can pick that up straight away. But if someone's having a private phone conversation and they're speaking we'd just hear a mumble.

Finally, staff also indicated that the presence of children in the MBU led to safety rules which did not mirror the ways in which mothers and families utilize space in their home, as we mentioned in chapter 4. An example of this was rules concerning the use of the kitchen, as noted by Joan:

> So you're not allowed to have babies in the kitchen or the milk room. In the past, years ago there was—obviously at home people do it differently—but in a hospital, even staff can't take babies in there. Years ago there was a baby burnt with hot water on the leg. And the other good thing about—that was sometimes an issue for a mum like, the baby's unsettled, they want to go in and make the baby's bottle if they're bottle fed or make themselves a cup of coffee they can't take the baby in.

Such rules were perceived to limit the movement of service users in the MBU, and had the potential to affect the ways in which they spent time with their babies and children—creating potential challenges to one of the functions of the MBU in terms of preparing mothers to return home and to care for their babies and children. However, Joan went on to note that, for this purpose built MBU, there were at least alternatives available:

> you might have noticed now in the dining room area as well as the main kitchen area, which has got the toddler proof gate thing, across on the other side there's a kitchen sink with a fridge. And so I think that area means that mums can still be with the baby and get themselves a drink or cereal or cheese and biscuits without having to take the baby to the kitchen. So that area works reasonably well I think.

Overall, there were evident tensions in both the design of the physical space and the rules within it in terms of the ability for an institutional space to approximate home for service users.

SMOKING

Staff identified smoking as a key concern within the MBU, both in terms of the physical design of the MBU and the rules within it as a health institution, saying that it was a "huge issue" (Alannah) and "the bane of our existence" (Brie). Smoking was not allowed in the MBU nor on its grounds, although there were places people smoked around the perimeter. Service users were encouraged to give up smoking when they arrived, with free nicotine patches and support available. Interestingly, staff had differences of opinion in relation to whether service users should give up smoking when they arrived at the MBU. For example, Alannah said:

> we had our morning community meeting today, and our head nurse said "It's a good time to give up smoking." Meaning that, you know, you can get free nicotine patches and support to do it. But it's also, when you've just had a baby, or you've just had a severe mental health issue, it's probably not the day to give up smoking for people. So, you know, even though in an ideal world people wouldn't smoke, and as a health organisation we should promote not smoking—but the reality is people smoke. And some of the people we have sometimes have chronic mental health issues and they do tend to smoke more and it's harder to shift.

Brie similarly indicated that perhaps it was important to be pragmatic about smoking and to ensure the safety of both staff and service users, while also noting that it was "the best time in their life" to stop given the fact that they had just had a baby:

> At the end of the day I would say to my staff, if you've got someone totally agitated, screaming, give me a—where they're involuntary and you can't at night

> go out and escort them, it's too unsafe, it's dark, it's all of those things—I don't care as long as you make it unobtrusive and in one of the corners of—like, I don't want staff to put themselves at risk. We talk about smoking, look, it's the best time in their life to give up smoking. Now, I smoked for many years and I understand the addiction type thing but there are certain places that they can go to. We will always offer them patches, inhalers, all of those things for free if they want to take them up. And it's an occasional problem.

In general, most staff agreed that it was not in the interests of very unwell or agitated service users to be required to give up smoking. However, other staff viewed smoking more negatively, and took a harder stance against smoking by service users, with Josie saying that it was "not okay" to elect to smoke in "secret hidey holes," noting that "it's a nice environment—people get really angsty about smokers being around their children." She went on to say that there would also be issues if smoking was allowed, particularly due to the presence of babies on site: "And if you were at a ward where smoking was allowed close by, what would happen is people would come back smelling like smoke strongly and then interact with the babies because that's what—and that's not okay." Joan similarly discussed issues of smoking around babies, noting both the necessity of not smoking around other people's babies and asking service users to "prioritize" their own babies over smoking:

> We ask mum to prioritise the babies when they want to go out for a smoke because we encourage them not to take the babies and smoke around the babies. But that if they want to go for a smoke like, if the baby's asleep that's fine, but if the baby's needing a feed we'd say you need to feed the baby before you go for a smoke, that's a bit of an issue.

Regardless of their views on smoking, all staff agreed that smoking posed a "huge architectural issue" (Alannah) due to the challenge of finding a spot away from other service users and their babies and children, but also close enough for those service users who did smoke to access the area easily and safely. She noted: "You can't have it [a designated smoking spot] somewhere where other people are going to be exposed—especially with babies. So how you design that, like where you would have it, I don't know. But surely there's a spot not too far away."

All staff indicated that, regardless of their views on smoking and the challenges of finding an appropriate place, it was ultimately important to have a designated spot for smoking, and that this was an important design consideration for purpose built MBUs. For example, Josie said that "it would have been nicer if there was some declared smoking areas before we moved so that it could be policed well." Staff said that the lack of a clear designated smoking area on the site (rather than around the perimeter) led to numerous issues, including the messy nature of having butts spread around when people smoked secretly in hidden places on the site, such as service entrances. For example, Brie said: “My biggest issue that I bang on about is butts around the front door. I don’t want to see them. If they can take a little bit of alfoil and put it in the bin please. I can’t stand a service entrance where I’m picking up butts.”

Alannah went on to say that having a smoking area that “mixed” service users from the MBU with other units was also problematic: “Sometimes we have some vulnerable young women that it’s not the best that they’re mixing with other patients. So the fact that we can’t have a designated smoking area for ourselves I think is an issue.”

Other staff also noted safety concerns for service users leaving the site to smoke at night in particular, with Brie saying:

> And I worry about safety and security of our young women, particularly at night in the dark. I’ve got a duty of care and if anything happened to one of those women who’d be responsible in the coroner’s court? I don’t want to have to test that but I think you make all these rules and they’re insisting to go out into the dark and someone, whatever, it concerns me particularly when they’re supposed to go out to the perimeter of the hospital. That’s a long way in the dark and pretty unsafe. And we’re trying to treat people with a less restrictive manner now so we don’t want to say, you can’t do this and you can’t do that. However, we have to worry about their safety.

Joan similarly pointed to safety issues with leaving the MBU at night, including after the doors were locked and detained/sectioned service users would have to be escorted to a place outside to smoke, leading to challenges with staffing inside the MBU:

> And there’s a bit behind us so basically there are designated smoking spots. So there’s one over the back but they’re all like—I don’t know what the closest would be, I’m not very good at distance—maybe 100 metres from the entrance, exit. So that’s okay in the daytime and it’s more of an issue at night time so we don’t like the mums going out once it’s dark to smoke and certainly from a certain time of the night which I should go, no. I think it’s 10:00, yeah, the doors get locked and then no one can go out. So it is an issue, particularly when you’ve got someone who’s maybe particularly—and the other issue for nursing staff is if someone is detained also that it’s not safe for them to go out by themselves, they have to be escorted. And then there’s a question of, is it fair to ask nursing staff to be sort of passively smoking and stuff like that. So that certainly is a big issue.

Joan also highlighted her concerns about passive smoking when staff had to escort service users, mirroring the concerns noted above about smoking around babies in the MBU. Issues of staffing and safety were also noted by Farida, who said that staff had to "naughtily" find alternative ways for service users to smoke at nighttime when it wasn't possible to have a staff member walk with them outside:

> It's a legal drug, you can tell people it's not good for them but you can't say—you can say you can't smoke on hospital grounds but there's that space over by the tree which isn't considered to be part of the health service so you're allowed to smoke there. But it's not easy distance and especially what we tend to do on night duty is very naughtily give them a little bit of Alfoil [aluminium foil] to put their buts in and just get them to smoke out the front of the building. Because there's only two of us on nights you can't spare a staff member to go out of the ward for even 10 minutes and leave somebody else there by themselves with a minimum of six babies and five other mums. And I'm not having them go out by themselves to walk to where a designated smoking spot is because it's just not safe.

In general, while staff held varying views about the extent to which service users should be encouraged to give up smoking when they were admitted, all staff agreed that smoking was a key consideration in the design of MBUs. Service users' safety—particularly given that all were women—was particularly important in this regard, with staff indicating that there needed to be a close, policed, private space for service users to smoke, which could also be well maintained. However, staff also agreed that smoking was problematic around babies in particular and that other service users who did not smoke could be upset by the presence of other people smelling of smoke near their babies and children. Some staff felt that service users should not have the opportunity to smoke after being admitted—effectively requiring them to give up smoking. However, previous research has noted that this may be counter to service user well-being, leading to stress (Shepley et al. 2017), and therefore smoking should be accommodated within mental health units—for example, through the use of smoking rooms. Michele Crossley (2000) has similarly argued that the focus on reducing "risky" behaviors in health policies is often limited and naïve, offering only a narrow view of the complexities of people's health, which often overlooks the importance of identity and autonomy. These issues clearly come to the fore in policies within units such as Park House and mirror tensions noted in previous chapters between autonomy and institutional policies. Overall, then, smoking was a key challenge in the design of the MBU, representing many of the competing challenges in designing a safe institutional space that met competing needs for staff and service users and their children.

NOISE

Another key issue of concern in terms of the design of the MBU was noise. Like smoking, noise highlighted the potential for strain between the communal, institutional, and therapeutic uses of the space in the MBU, although some aspects of noise were inevitable, as Alannah said:

> It can be loud when babies are crying and stuff and they will . . . the rooms are not totally soundproof, so they will wake up other babies, other mums. I think that . . . what are you going to do? It can be an issue when there's toddlers as well, who can be a bit louder even and more mobile.

While, as Alannah indicates, crying babies or toddlers are an unavoidable element of noise in an MBU, there were particular design concerns present that related to noise and that staff felt could have been avoided through different design choices. Brie highlighted this in the extract below:

> And I mean that's my experience in any architectural-built hospital around Australia is that they don't actually understand screaming, distressed, unregulated babies and how distressing that noise is and how, with no carpet and all that sort of thing around to buffer that nose, that it sort of travels. And so we never have enough night spaces to put babies so that they're not waking people. And that's disappointing because we couldn't have been clearer about some of our experiences [in the planning stage consultations]. And I certainly had to do night duty one night and we had two 17 month old twins who basically screamed in blood curdling screams so that people 70 feet away were complaining about the noise. And they could do it for six and a half hours straight.

Brie indicated that the design of the MBU created particular challenges for design, particularly in relation to places for babies to be at nighttime; an issue raised frequently by service users themselves, as seen in the following chapter. In addition to places for babies to sleep, staff indicated that issues of soundproofing had been mixed up by the architects, such that some places were soundproofed appropriately, and others weren't. In particular, staff noted that the soundproofing of the nurseries created issues, as discussed by Constance:

> The soundproofing, they really got the idea of why we wanted things soundproofed and not soundproofed wrong. So initially when we had the babies in the nursery you couldn't hear them anywhere. So all the nurseries are soundproof, awesome. And in the nurses' station there's a little monitor. The nurses' station is also soundproofed right. Initially there was a little monitor

> where you could look and see the red line and that could tell that someone was crying but you couldn't hear them. So now at least you can hear in the nurses' station but if you step out of the nurses' station you can't actually hear the babies crying.

Problems with soundproofing such that staff and service users couldn't hear babies crying in the nursery unless they were in the nurses' station where the baby monitors are were also highlighted by Hannah. She also indicated that the soundproofing of the nurses' station led to other issues, including hearing phones ringing and checks from security:

> You definitely can't hear the phones, you can't hear the walkie talkie when the security check in morning and night that you're alive and kicking. So unless you're actually physically in the office [nurses' station] you can't hear any of that, you can't hear the babies in the nurseries. So while they did a really good job on the soundproofing [of the nurseries] so other people aren't disturbed by the babies crying, unless you're actually in the office where the intercoms are hardwired up to, you can't hear the babies crying. And because there's only two of us on a night duty and it happens during the day when I'm in there, the nurses haven't got time to sit in the office and the office is not well designed. That's probably one of the areas that isn't well designed. Unless you're actually there then you tend to miss the phone calls and you miss hearing what's going on in the nurseries and the rooms.

Other issues of design related to the placement of televisions, which numerous staff raised as an issue of concern. There are three televisions within the main spaces where service users spend time, and these were often on, including at times when the researchers were present, as noted in chapter 4. This created a noisy environment in addition to people talking, and staff also indicated that they perceived this to be negative for mental health and the development of babies. For example, Diana said:

> And also within that space there are three televisions: so one in the lounge, one in the main area [dining area] and then, ridiculously, one in the play pen area where the babies are. And that one doesn't get turned on very often in the day but the other two are constantly on and it just creates more noise. And I don't think that's helpful for the patients having that background noise. And they're certainly not going to feel like that's their right to turn it off I wouldn't have thought. So I think it's hard for the clients then. I think it's sometimes hard for the staff to turn the TVs off because you'd have to then ask everyone, is it okay if I turn this off because you don't know who is actually watching it or whether it's just been on in the background.

Later, Diana indicated that not only were the televisions problematic for noise and mental health, but also potentially for relationships between service users themselves and also service users and staff, in that they could be a source of tension if some people wanted to watch while others did not. In general, however, there were concerns that televisions created a noisy environment that was not conducive to mental well-being.

Other staff also had concerns about noise and mental health, including in relation to overcrowding in small spaces which did not easily accommodate staff, service users, and babies and children. For example, Alannah said that noise was something that staff needed to be "aware of," given that it might be overwhelming to some service users:

> We have ward round, so we all meet, it's a huge amount of people, sometimes too many I think, and we talk about plans for everyone. And I've noticed we'll rush into that common area, the kitchen/dining, and people will be talking to patients about stuff. But it's really loud—and it's really, you know, sometimes I think those conversations need to be taken off somewhere a bit more private. But just so that, the volume in that room and the movement and the activity level isn't so high because that, I think, is detrimental sometimes for people's mental health. It feels quite overwhelming. Even as a staff member sometimes. There's just too much going on.

Similar issues of noise, overcrowding and design were also raised by staff in relation to the location of the nurseries, laundries, and visitors' toilets. These were located close to each other and caused issues of crowding and noise in the nurseries, also noted by service users in the following chapter. For example, Josie responded to a question about noise by saying:

> Yes, and anyone who was thinking wisely would not put the laundries across from the nurseries or the toilets and the bathrooms across from the nursery . . . we ask visitors to not go past the door by the nurseries but the visitors' toilets are past there. If they'd thought that through it would have been nice to have the visitors' toilet in a place that wasn't so intrusive to the patient care. Because some people have some odd visitors and if your baby is in Nursery 1 and you think so and so's drunk boyfriend's here and going to the bathroom and it's across the hallway from where your baby is sleeping and you can't see that from where you're sitting, that could be quite anxiety provoking.

Noise was also an issue in terms of alarms, with the testing of alarms often waking babies, as Joan said:

> I think the habit of checking the alarms regularly, the duress and fire alarms, particularly Monday morning about 10:30 when everyone's babies are down

> for a nap. This week one of the girls [mothers], her little girl went down—her baby is 10 months—had been down for 10 minutes before the alarm went off so woke up and wouldn't go back. So that was a 10 o'clock nap. And then her 2 o'clock one there was another alarm testing and it woke her up. And then another day that happened to her as well, you know, that's too much. They need to be respectful of that.

Here, the issue of noise and the requirements of the unit—checking alarms—clearly conflicted with the needs of service users and their babies and children.

Noise was also discussed by staff as problematic in relation to small elements of design which nevertheless had big effects on people's experiences of the MBU, and again highlights strains between creating a homely environment as well as one which met the demands of an institutional environment. An example of this was the doors, which nearly all people interviewed raised as problematic, and as we discussed in chapters 3 and 4. For example, Brie noted that the noise made by doors was especially a problem for the particular group of service users in the MBU who were unlikely to sleep well anyway, such that small noises would be likely to break their sleep. Similarly, Farida also discussed the noise made by the doors:

> We check they've got husbands and partners staying otherwise we wake them up every three-quarters of an hour or hour or whenever we do rounds because using the opener swipe thing it gives a real heavy click to disengage. And then you've got the door going when you open it too. So we end up putting face washers or towels over the doors to stop them going shut. It's lovely that they close so that people aren't as—you've got a lot more safety around personal possessions during the day. But it's so noisy that you just cannot have those doors shut at night and be able to—it would be nice if you could say, yep, go to bed, I'll see you in 12 hours. But duty of care and you go and check at least hourly if not more often and so the rooms have got to be open.

Overall noise was evidently a key concern for staff. As Josie said: "It would be nicer if they'd thought of, actually what it means to have a mum, a dad, and a baby in a room and a worker and probably two workers." There was a general feeling that issues of noise had not been adequately considered in the design of the unit, and that in particular the needs of a space accommodating both adults with particular mental health needs and children had not been met.

ACCOMMODATING CHILDREN IN A MOTHER-BABY UNIT

While the space was generally considered homely by the staff (with associated tensions of an institution approximating homeliness as outlined throughout this chapter), participants highlighted interesting issues in relation to the ability to accommodate children of different ages within the same space. As in the case of noise, there was agreement among staff that—while specifically meant to be a unit that included children—children were not well catered for at least in some respects. A key example of this was the number of nurseries available as noted previously. While Park House could accommodate six mothers, there was only three nurseries, leading to babies sleeping in a range of rooms, which some staff members indicated was an issue. Alannah said:

> So a lot of rooms get used to put babies in. Because we've got six bedrooms but not all mums . . . the idea is that the babies will be in with mums and they look after their babies, but sometimes they're too unwell to do that and need to build up to doing that. And so we've got three nurseries, but that's only half of the number of people that are admitted here, so that multipurpose room will have babies in it, the group room will have babies in it, I think sometimes that Registrar office will have babies, the loungeroom.

Joan also discussed space and babies, highlighting particularly the fact that it was likely that service users may prefer to have their babies elsewhere or cared for by staff so that they could sleep:

> Some people want their baby in the room no matter what, some people don't want the baby anywhere near them sort of thing. And we tend to get more of the ones who don't want the babies near them rather than the ones who want the babies with them all the time. And even if often when they first come in they might—understandably I would be reluctant to hand the baby over to strangers because staff are initially strangers—but once they've settled in here they tend to like to have them looked after once they realise we're trustworthy. So nurseries and particularly at night and more particularly sleep is really important in terms of getting well. So when mums are first admitted the night staff tend to look after the babies and then as the mums get better we encourage them to do more of the overnight care. So where babies sleep can be hotly contested because usually you can only have one baby in the nursery. Sometimes with the really tiny little babies you can have more than one in a nursery but most of that like, old ones wake each other up. So three nurseries you've got three babies there so often that handover room is used.

Interestingly, the flip side of the availability of nurseries was also noted by Joan, who said that "the option of the nursery can contribute to mum's avoidance of the baby I guess," while also saying "but there are also lots of opportunities both inside and outside to be together." In this way, nurseries embodied some of the challenges of the MBU and its design, with sometimes competing demands around the needs of service users and staff. Nevertheless, the fact that there were not enough nurseries was continually mentioned by both staff and service users (see following chapter) as a key limitation to the design of the unit.

Another key design issue in relation to children discussed by staff related to the play spaces inside the main living/dining area. Staff also noted that the play spaces weren't designed appropriately, and that this was directly counter to what staff had asked for in the consultation process. For example, Farida said:

> So one of the things that was really important for us was to have the corrals for the babies to be in so that if mums needed to make something in the kitchen they could pop the baby in the corral and the baby could be safe. And we asked for them to be glass sided so that the babies could see out. But the way they're positioned it means that the babies can't see in the kitchen. And they did coloured glass so the babies can't see through it.

Brie said that this was a specific example of the design of the unit not taking into account consultation with staff, saying "it was like talking to bricks" and that

> sometimes they did pretty things rather than practical. Because they had these little thoughts in their mind about, this would be really pretty. Costs lots of money but—and I'll give you an example. In our little corral where we can separate our babies from our toddlers for safety they actually made them solid glass, pretty glass so the babies couldn't actually see their parents through. And they just didn't understand, they were really upset that I made them take the non-see through glass out. They had no concept that if a baby can't see you you're not there. So just part of the issue in the build was they didn't actually come back and ask the practical people to go through. They allowed executive—three layers above me—to sign off.

In this way the baby corrals clearly represented issues with the design of the unit as one that needed to accommodate the needs of mothers and babies, with staff indicating that the architects did not understand the developmental needs of children and as such did not take these into account in their design of some spaces. Another example of this was the need to store or facilitate the numerous equipment needed by babies and children such as cots, highchairs, and prams. Hannah mentioned this, noting that it was particularly problematic because the space needed to be flexible depending on whether there were six newborns or six toddlers, or a mixture of ages:

> We need child seats, we need different size pushers and prams and things because we have different size babies. Like, if we have six babies that are under 3 months we need different equipment than if we have five babies that are over 12 months old. And they do come in blobs like, we might have a whole lot of weenie ones. Like right at this moment we've got three babies that are under 5 weeks' old. But the week before last we would have had all babies over 10 months. So that's different. Yeah, because we've got to have different prams. Like, you know the sort of pram a toddler is in is different to a newborn so we have to have six of each, child seats, and highchairs. There's no obvious storing spot for the highchairs in the dining area. And you know what toddlers are like in eating, they're disgusting. The place where the piano is I don't know why they didn't consider that to be a highchair storage area. We need a highchair storage area and we need those little booster seats for the chairs.

Josie similarly discussed the issue of equipment and space, noting that in addition to service users and their children there were often also partners or other family members present in spaces:

> Also the dining area is way too small. Because we have highchairs and we have pushers and we have dining tables we take a lot more space than six patients normally would. Because we're never six patients, we're 12 patients and then we've often got other family members. And our patients need a lot of equipment like, six of them need highchairs or prams. So if you're rocking a pram at a dining table you actually need a lot more room than if you're sitting there by yourself. So that area is a little bit small for the purpose.

As such staff highlighted that the functional needs of babies and children were not well accommodated for within the space, with a lack of design consideration for the types of activities that are required when children are present, such as rocking a pram. Another key example of this was the fact that there was no toddler toilet, despite the frequent presence of toddlers in the unit. Mathilde articulated this, saying "We needed a toddler toilet, we got a disabled toilet, and we didn't get a toddler toilet. We wanted to be set up more to be young child friendly," while Joan said: "And I mean I had a real issue in that I understand we've got to meet disability regulations and got no problems with that whatsoever, but we already had two disabled bedrooms and a disabled toilet. It wouldn't allow our bathroom, which is largely a children's bathroom, to have a toddler toilet which we'd always had."

Finally, staff indicated that design was challenging in relation to the range of ages in the babies and toddlers who were with their mothers in the unit, saying that this created some challenges in relation to activities and use of spaces. For example, again in relation to the corral, Diana said:

> And a toddler certainly gets to the stage very quickly where they want to get out. It's just too tiny an area so that could have been utilised a bit better than what it was. And that's the balance too because we have the age groups from newborns up to 2 so you've got toddlers running around and you've got vulnerable babies and that's trying to get the balance of keeping them both safe without being too constrictive on the toddlers.

Josie agreed with this, saying she "could see why other mother-baby units sort of cut it off when babies are mobile," and that while she didn't think this was necessarily good policy, she "can see from a practical design point" that having children of various ages in the same unit was very challenging.

In general, staff felt that there were a range of issues in the unit which did not cater well to babies and children, an interesting conflict given the purpose of Park House. Staff generally expressed concerns that their requests were not taken into account in designing the unit and the space within it, creating a range of small issues that they felt affect the experience of service users.

FLEXIBLE OUTDOOR SPACES FACILITATE PARENT–CHILD RELATIONSHIPS

While there were issues with accommodating children of different ages in the MBU, one space which was consistently highlighted as facilitating parent (mother)-child relationships was the two outdoor courtyards. These spaces were generally spoken of in positive ways by staff, with participants noting that they were well designed and allowed for positive interactions between mothers and their children. For example, Joan told a story about flexible play in the courtyard between mothers and their babies playing with the sand table and "doing a little playgroup out there," going on to say "and so that sort of thing can happen which is good." Similarly, Constance said:

> Also having the two outdoor areas, where you can go with your baby or with your toddler and have a bit of a roam around and sit in the outside area. I mean I thought last week it was pretty sensational to see three of our mums in a

> splashing pool with their three babies and they're [the babies are] all naked, blowing bubbles and giggling, and I can't say that I've ever seen that on another ward.

The inclusion of outdoor spaces in mental health units, including MBUs units, has been discussed in previous literature, with researchers noting that outdoor spaces are typically seen by staff and service users as promoting positive mental health outcomes (Shepley et al. 2017). As such, the design of Park House with the two courtyard spaces offers positive avenues to mental health improvements, both directly (e.g., through exposure to nature elements) and more indirectly (e.g., by offering opportunities to build relationships between mothers and their babies or children). However, staff did note that there were some issues—especially in relation to the slide, which was made of metal—an issue which staff again attributed to oversight on the part of the design team. Josie explained:

> There's been a lot of grizzling [by service users] about the metal slippery dip underneath, being in the full sun. And being able to see . . . you bring your three year old in, you can see that playground from almost every part of this hospital. If you're three you want to be on that playground if you can see it. If it's 40 degrees and it's only 20 inside here you cannot understand why you can't be playing on that playground. And for it to be a metal one in full sun and the soft fall at the bottom, because it's so dark coloured that gets really hot too and on really hot days it's not safe to go outside if you're little.

Again, here Josie highlighted a discrepancy between the needs of the MBU—to accommodate children—and a lack of foresight in relation to design. Overall however, staff noted the outside spaces were a particularly positive component of the unit which allowed for a range of activities that met the needs of people in the unit.

CONCLUDING THOUGHTS

While staff were generally positive about the design of Park House, they indicated a broad range of issues with the space and the way it functioned as both institution and "home." In particular, there was a general feeling that the space did not specifically meet the needs of service users—particularly children—which was particularly interesting given that Park House was a purpose built unit. As Brie said "if I say that this is better than we've ever had, however, if I was honest, it comes with its own set of problems in that they didn't quite understand the brief for our clients." In particular, and reflecting both previous chapters and the perspectives of service users in the following chapter, there were evident tensions in the design of the space in terms of its ability to create a sense of home and provide privacy, while also performing the functions required of it as an institution. This is reflective of research by Novotná and colleagues (2011, 1532), who found "tensions in maintaining a safe therapeutic environment that was simultaneously supportive of client autonomy." Moreover, issues in meeting the needs of children—and therefore being able to promote relationships between mothers and their children—were also identified by staff.

One particularly positive aspect of the space identified by staff was that of the outside spaces, which they saw as facilitating of mother-baby relationships and as able to promote positive mental health outcomes. Interestingly, this stands somewhat in contrast to our own observations of these outdoor spaces as noted in chapter 4, which identified the boundaries of these garden areas to function as a panopticon, promoting regulation and management of service users. This was not an issue brought up by staff, which perhaps provides insight into the different perspectives we bring as researchers and observers, highlighting the importance of acknowledging the situated nature of the different points of view discussed within this book. Service users similarly brought their own views of the outdoor spaces, as well as the rest of Park House, and these are outlined further in the following chapter.

Chapter 6

The Therapeutic Space

Service User Perspectives

As noted in chapter 2, there is a small body of literature that has considered service users' experiences of MBUs. This literature tends to show relatively high levels of satisfaction and a preference for MBUs over other types of psychiatric units (Antonysamy, Wieck, and Wittkowski 2009; Nair et al. 2010; Neil, Sanderson, and Wieck 2006). None of the previous literature that has included the experiences of women admitted to an MBU, however, has considered space and its potential effect on their time in the unit. In this chapter we outline the views and experiences of service users with respect to the space at Park House. As with the previous interviews and ethnographic data collection outlined in the preceding chapters, our interview questions with service users oriented toward exploring perceptions of the space, with a particular focus on noise, privacy, and light. We were also interested in how these elements interacted with or were balanced in service users' accounts with their own personal needs—particularly those of their relationship with their baby or toddler who was admitted with them, their relationships more broadly, and their mental health needs.

Interviews were conducted with service users after consultation with staff, and following ethical considerations particularly concerning genuine informed consent (Marzano 2007). As such, interviews took a variety of shapes and forms. Overall, they were semi-structured and open-ended, with key questions concerning noise, privacy, light, safety, and space use. Mothers were the primary service users, so we focused our attention on them, including individual interviews and group interviews, as noted in chapter 2. However, interviews were sometimes conducted with (or in the presence of) their partners, and, in one case, with a mother-in-law. Babies and toddlers were almost always present. As such, interviews here represented the accounts of service users' experiences, but also often *demonstrations of* their experience—the interviewer was taken to locations in Park House where issues could be demonstrated, and in these spaces talk often oriented to what babies or toddlers were doing in the moment, and service users discussed issues among themselves while also interacting with the interviewer. Therefore, while thirteen service users (ten mothers, two fathers, and one mother-in-law) ultimately participated in interviews in one form or another, the data that form the basis of this chapter are drawn not only from their textual accounts, but also from observation and illustrations of their interactions with each other and the space in the unit.

As in chapter 5, we followed Braun and Clarke's (2006, 2013) approach to thematic analysis to explore the data. This chapter is divided into four themes— Homeliness; Tensions Concerning Privacy: Isolation, Security, and Assistance; Spaces Facilitating Relationships; and Spaces for Sleep as Less than Ideal. As in the previous chapters, all participants were provided with pseudonyms and other identifying information has been removed from the data extracts included here.

HOMELINESS

As noted throughout this book, one of the key features of Park House is the attempts made at homeliness in the design of the unit. For example, the ambiguities of homely and clinical space sit uncomfortably beside each other when the symbolic and material dimensions of home versus institution hang in balance. Almost all service users discussed this aspect, noting, for example, as Sarah did, that: "This doesn't even look like a hospital ward, really *(laughs)*, it's just like a house." For service users this aspect of Park House appeared to be important, both in terms of their subjective experience while staying there and in terms of their ability to have family visit or partners and older children stay. Often, service users noted small features of their rooms or the broader space that made them feel "at home," as in Beth's discussion of her room:

Beth: And the little alcove in there to put your stuff on, the other rooms didn't have like anywhere to put your shower bits umm . . . and . . . I love that there's . . . I haven't used it yet but there's like a book nook. Like next to the desk area there's like a cushion right in front of the windows . . .
Interviewer: So you're going to use that? When you get round to it?
Beth: Yep that's one of . . . I've always wanted a book nook *(laughs)* so . . . *(laughs a bit more)*

Homeliness here was often discussed in relation to spaces as being "inviting"—here seen in the small features of Beth's space that made her enjoy and feel comfortable within it.

In other accounts, elements of homeliness (or interruptions to homeliness) were noted in relation to light, openness, and noise. Light and openness were key features of the space that were highlighted as important by service users. In particular, service users focused on natural rather than artificial light, and the feeling of space as open and friendly. For example, in response to questions about the space, and from two separate interviews, Sarah and Nathan (a father staying at the time of interviews) said:

Nathan: It's bright and it's open and it's, you know, there's space and you're not in everyone's way all the time and you can do your own thing and the lounge room looks inviting and the bedroom look inviting and the hallways are I don't know, they're designed, it just looks more open and friendly . . . I find the open area, the dining area and lounges, they're quite friendly, very large amount of light in there which is great. So they're . . . that's a very nice space . . . Having light which wasn't too harsh—which was "homely"—was also important for babies and toddlers, particularly in relation to sleep:

Sarah: In all of the rooms, you don't even need to have the light on during the day because there's plenty of you know like the windows . . .

Interviewer: Natural light?

Sarah: Yeah, yeah.

Interviewer: And how do you like that?

Sarah: I do, I do. [Child's name] likes it as well, she sleeps a lot better at nighttime because she sleeps in here [multi-purpose interview room] and these window blinds are open and there's enough light coming in from outside.

Interviewer: Ah, okay, so that natural light is important for you.

Sarah: It is, because you know you—when you're stuck in a hospital ward and all there are these fluorescent yellow lights, it's really stressful and I feel very trapped, very . . . yeah I need open windows [blinds] and stuff.

Interestingly, perhaps due to this focus on homeliness, service users also frequently discussed practical elements of the space which were seen as problematic. These issues can be read as concerns which interfere with the homeliness of the space, or the ability for service users to feel as though they were "at home." One key concern in this regard was the temperature of the ward, which we were told was set at 24 degrees Celsius through a central unit, and which several of the participants indicated was too hot. When asked to reflect on the space, Sarah said: "It's really hot all the time in here, but I don't know if it's the way the temperature is set to 24 or whatever but it's always stuffy in here, constantly. You can't open the windows, you can only open the blinds."

At times the issue of the temperature was discussed in relation to functionality, bringing the concern back to service users' mental health rather than their subjective experience of being "at home" in the unit (although of course these two concerns are intertwined). Leanne, for example, noted: "It's awful, awfully hot in here all the time—it's set at 24 degrees I think umm but it's always so hot. I've got the fan going 24/7 in my room . . . I don't know why it's centrally controlled to 24 there's obviously a reason but not all of us cope at that . . . can function very well at that."

Not all design-related issues brought up by service users focused solely on homely aspects, however, since ultimately the purpose of Park House as an MBU meant that design elements had to include catering for women, their babies and toddlers, and sometimes their partners, other children, and visiting family members. As such, practical issues related to sharing the space with other people were a feature of service users' interviews and discussion of the space. An example of this is in Anne's discussion below of the width of the corridors:

Anne: The design, to give it a negative point, the ways are not wide enough.
Interviewer: OK so the corridors?
Anne: The corridors are not wide enough because we have to go sometime with the pram there, and sometime come two prams and it's just enough and if you go here it's all in the foot room it's not big enough.
Interviewer: So not big enough for prams to go past each other?
Anne: Yeah, or even with one it's sometimes a problem if another person . . . if another person comes especially at the corners.

Noise also featured in service users' accounts of the space as shared with other mothers and their children. Noise was particularly problematic in terms of interrupted sleep, and the corresponding interference with bonding and recovery. Beth noted:

> The bedrooms aren't soundproofed quite enough, I don't think, like you can hear other people outside and in the corridor and that wakes my son up. Umm and the same with the windows umm the blinds aren't any like black out blinds or something like that in there if the baby's going to be in the bedrooms cos he wakes up at 5 o'clock every morning when the sun comes up umm . . . *(sigh)* and doesn't settle well in the evenings as well. But *(sigh)* but I mean that's just . . . small things.

Melissa also commented on noise in relation to her baby's sleep, noting that noise issues had the potential to wake her baby, and the solution was to compromise on privacy:

> the doors are so loud to open and close you have to like hang a towel 'cos if your baby's sleeping the doors are so loud that if you open the door it would wake

> them up so you have to like kind of hang a towel there so your door's never like fully to kind of, so it's never fully closed, so yeah . . . I think that's the only thing with privacy that's a bit difficult.

Service users also highlighted concerns that they might wake up other people while caring for their crying babies in the night, highlighting particular elements of the design (such as distance between bedrooms and spaces to prepare bottles), as problematic in this regard. Anne said: "And there *(points)* where you can make the milk is sometime the ways are extremely long. Maybe if you had to build two small rooms to make milk up it would be maybe smarter, because you have to go so long with your crying baby, you wake other people." For others, noise wasn't seen as an issue. Sarah indicated: "It's also really quiet . . . the way all the doors open and close so they can block off the nurseries and the babies are quiet and she comes and sleeps in here [in the interview room] at night time so I get sleep in my room." And Nina (a mother-in-law boarding at Park House while her daughter-in-law was admitted with her baby) also noted:

> It's funny because I'm usually a person that gets quite umm I don't sleep with noise and stuff like that and I don't know if it's because I've been looking after my grand-daughter and sleeping with white noise and everything . . . the noise hasn't really been bothering me like the doors in our bedrooms are really quite soundproof so once you shut the door you can just vaguely hear noises occasionally, yeah the bedroom area is a quite quiet so I'm a bit impressed with that.

Service users' different experiences with noise may reflect differences in tolerance for noise levels of locations in different parts of the ward. For example, Sarah's older toddler was sleeping separately to her in an interview room, while Beth's baby was spending at least some of the time sleeping in her room with her, meaning that any noise which woke him also woke her. Overall, however, noise appeared to be a factor in interrupting the sense of homeliness of Park House, whether it was due to the fact that service users could hear others, were afraid of making noise themselves, or were surprised at the lack of noise in the unit.

TENSIONS CONCERNING PRIVACY: ISOLATION, SECURITY, AND ASSISTANCE

As seen in the accounts of Nina and Melissa above, concerns about noise were often related to concerns about privacy because noise affected people's ability to keep their bedroom doors closed or open. Overall, privacy was a key concern to people who were interviewed. Anne discussed this: "Privacy is very important and I'm thinking that sometimes there's too much the doors open, too much the rooms are stuck together so where I live in rooms number 1 and 2 you lie awake there there's somebody crying you hear everything, so for me it's like sleepless, it's not that nice."

In this sense, then, being able to hear others around you, particularly when they are distressed, encroached on feelings of being "at home" in the ward. Interestingly, however, and as we discuss later in this section, communal spaces and shared experiences with other mothers were typically discussed as helpful in dealing with mental health concerns, and thus the extent to which feeling a sense of homeliness in the ward could only go so far.

Indeed, a key theme in interviews was the tension between feeling a sense of privacy while also feeling secure and safe, but not isolated. There is a delicate balance between a fear of isolation and a need to be private. Anne's words reflect these tensions: "[Privacy is] important when I am not that well. I feel isolated, or I feel watched. I think this is in our condition. It's very important."

Service users who identified more as "private people" noted that they wanted to stay in their bedrooms rather than use communal spaces. However, aspects of the space—whether intentional or not—meant that this was generally not possible. Connie said:

> When I'm feeling down I'll go back into my room umm but . . . I'm I try not to because I get more depressed so I think um it's probably a good thing that how the rooms are how they are because it kind of . . . it doesn't discourage them coming out but it does discourage them staying in.

In view of Connie's words regarding an encouragement to get out of their bedrooms and be with others, both the design and the routines facilitated socialization. In particular, mealtimes could be shared with all people staying at Park House and, as noted in chapter 4, baby facilities such as storing bottles and formula were at a distance from bedrooms, so there was no choice but to go there. Additionally, bedrooms did not contain leisure features such as televisions. Connie and her husband, Geoff (who was staying with her at the time of the interview) discussed this:

Connie: In the interests of . . . with mental health you're supposed to watch TV communally or . . . um . . . I certainly would have liked to have my own TV.

Interviewer: What do you think the impact of the design decisions has on privacy? You know there are a lot of clients and individuals. I guess that's different for everyone?

Geoff: Yeah I think you would benefit from a bit of that . . . in terms of atmosphere of what you'd like, you know, having a TV in your room but coming out if you needed to but just being around the communal areas you can't seem to have that . . . don't have your own space.

Conversely, other service users who were interviewed felt that the communal spaces such as kitchens and lounge areas were key to recovery because they promoted interactions with other mothers and a sense of "not being alone." Nathan (a father staying at the time of interviews) and Sarah (another mother) outline this in the extracts below:

Nathan: The main dining area there is also a bit of a common area so it's an opportunity for mothers to talk and get to know each other and they're all there which is great because all the women and the mothers that are here have usually got some form of uh depression or anxiety of something like that so I think it's very helpful that they talk amongst themselves which helps them *(sigh)* feel that they're not alone, you know . . . and, and um . . . a problem shared is a problem halved, so to speak. One gets . . .

Sarah: The shared spaces definitely help like we're all out in the lounge room in the night times and in the mornings we're all in the dining room area or talking to each other and it's an open space, it's not closed in and it doesn't feel like you're trapped and then the conversations would be a lot more . . . like you can just come and go whenever you want, umm and it also helps to have a lot of space for me and [child's name] to play together as well rather than being just stuck in a hospital room all the time.

Relatives and male partners also discussed their feeling that privacy needed to be balanced with ensuring that mothers interacted. For example, Nina (a mother-in-law staying in the unit with her daughter-in-law) noted in response to a question about the importance of personal privacy that

> [privacy is] very very important [to] my daughter-in-law at the moment—she is struggling with privacy so she's a very private person and where it doesn't bother me but for her, she, she really does appreciate her privacy umm the fact that the bedrooms are so far away from everything else actually makes a person who might be struggling, like my daughter-in-law is really struggling interacting with people, it actually forces her to interact with people, because she actually has to leave her bedroom to get everything because it's away from the room so I don't know whether that's been purposely done because sometimes when you're depressed you want to shut yourself away so as much as sometimes it's a pain having to come all the way all round to get the formula I think sometimes that it's been done on purpose because in the process you get to see different people on the way around and interact with people

Nina attempts to see things through the eyes and mind of her daughter-in-law, but as a family member she also has a degree of objectivity that her daughter-in-law may not have while unwell. She understands her daughter-in-law's nature as a "private person" and recognizes the added effort (on top of being depressed) that it takes for her to go out of her room. Nina continued:

> because to start with you know you think "Ah it's a pain in the bum, in the middle of the night, I've got to go aaaall the way around there to the formula room" and then you think "Ahhh" you know if we have a fridge in our room, we'd never have to leave our room so there'd be no interaction between the mum and the staff and only when staff needed to so I think, I think, yeah it's a good idea that there is distance between because it does actually physically get you up and walk[ing] around and yeah cos there's one umm consumer here that we very rarely see her and you think "ahh she must be struggling so much" and she might just be a private person but, you know, I just think I'd love to see her out and interacting more

Nina suggests that the absence of a fridge in the bedroom is deliberate. It is also unlikely that there would be a fridge in a mother's bedroom in her own home, further emphasizing the need to overcome the need to shut oneself off when unwell. Nina has the added benefit of noticing, and perhaps comparing, how other service users are managing.

In addition to finding a balance between privacy and isolation, other tensions were evident in interviews with respect to privacy and security. Balancing these potentially competing concerns has been a feature of our work with mental health units in the past (Authors 2012), and was also evident in interviews with service users at Park House. An example of this was provided again by Nina (mother-in-law):

> The staff are always very respectful of your privacy, they will always knock and, you know, ask permission to come in before they barge in and all the rest of it. But I do think that security probably has to be paramount especially when you've got little kids involved so um I think there's good privacy but yeah I think they have got a good balance.

Leanne also discussed this, saying: "Yeah, like I feel, I feel safe and I feel that my belongings are safe and that my own privacy is respected as well so . . . so it works well."

A final tension in considerations of privacy related to balancing privacy with getting help or assistance from staff. Often, overcoming this tension seemed to rely on staff awareness of service users' needs rather than particular aspects of the space itself. For example, Melissa said:

Melissa: I think it was very stand offish to start with because having to come to a place like this is very awfully confronting on many levels . . . admitting defeat one might say. So I really didn't know what to expect. So I had not real expectations, but after being here, I've been here 2 weeks nearly, I think and . . . I think that it's, I've got it working quite well the way I've got privacy but help is there just round the corner if I need it. Do you know what I mean?

Interviewer: Yeah.

Melissa: Like, I never feel like that my personal space is being invaded, invaded or anything like. But the nursing staff in particular have this uncanny ability to actually know when to appear almost appear out of nowhere.

While Melissa reflects positively on space and perhaps also how it might have contributed to the staff's ability to show up unobtrusively when required, other participants felt a sense of being observed; something which Anne in particular found hard to deal with:

> this place is made to watch me or to watch people so it's a bit difficult, I feel always a little bit two eyes are needed and sometimes too much watched. Everything sticks together and you see here even the people they watch and monitor can watch the people or can watch the floors or sometimes could give you that feeling that people they know everything, you know.

Overall, then, and especially in relation to the previous theme on homeliness, there were clearly some tensions and differences in service users' experiences of the space. These tensions were particularly evident at the juxtaposition between the space as needing to be clinical and desires for it to feel homely.

SPACES FACILITATING RELATIONSHIPS

While tensions were evident in the service users' discussions of privacy versus interacting with others and safety and security, many interview participants also noted that spaces which facilitated relationships—either with others in the unit or with their children—were important. For example:

Interviewer: What about mother-child interactions? Is this space designed to work for that?

Nathan: Yeah, yes there's quite opportunity there for mother-child interactions, you've got the lovely playgrounds there which is . . . when the weather gets a little bit bit better—it's not the best at the moment—umm it's a great opportunity for mum to get outside and interact with the child and there's a little, just behind the nurses' station there's a little, little, it's like a little infant pen which is you know another good space for mum to interact with her child.

Nathan's baby was only a few months old and was also their first child so perhaps he had more optimistic views of the play pen than others. Chapter 3 enlarges on the design problems of this area as a functional play space. Outdoor spaces, while subject to weather conditions and seasonal change, were mostly discussed as positive spaces that participants enjoyed being in with their children. The retractable shading facilitated weather constraints to some degree. Staff noted that it was retrofitted as a result of the weather and not always easy to operate. Nonetheless, Sarah also oriented to the outdoor spaces when thinking about where she could play with her toddler:

> She loves the playground and the gardens out there and the other thing about it which I didn't know until recently, if it rains or if it's too sunny or whatever there's like a like an automatic shade that goes over and then retracts again and it's a good help for her because I did . . . I did not want to take her outside I thought she'd get sunburnt and that helps.

Interestingly, in response to questions about relationships between mothers and their children, participants often focussed on spaces their *children* enjoyed being in, rather than spaces that theythemselves [as mothers] found therapeutic. However, participants' accounts varied widely in relation to the efficacy of the spaces in the unit in this regard. Indeed, overall, participants tended to feel that—apart from the outside space—the facilities were not appropriate for their baby or toddler regardless of their age. For example, Sarah, who had a walking toddler indicated that her child was often bored:

Interviewer: Just in terms of the space you know the way it's designed, how is it working for you? You know is there enough space for you and your child?
Sarah: Yeah I think it's more for me because she's the oldest here by a long shot, she has a lot of trouble, she finds that she's running round not knowing what to do a lot of the time.

Similarly, Beth, who had a toddler who was not yet walking, also said that there was not much for her child to do in the unit:

> I think that there needs to be more in the way of . . . for the younger like babies and stuff. Like I don't know how you would do that but there needs to be more design around that because obviously the older kids who are walking and that you can take outside and that and you know um . . . but I kind of just have to let my son crawl around but . . . I dunno even if an indoor playground or something would've been . . .

While Sarah and Beth had toddlers, Connie, who had a baby who was only a month old, reflected upon her spatial needs in terms of connecting with her baby:

Interviewer: Now your little one is small but how is the space designed for you to build your relationship with your child, how does the space help you connect?

Connie: Mmm he is very young . . . I don't really know. I think what they've done outside and that and even in the communal area the little play area, where they can go on the ground and put them on . . . pop them on . . . [play equipment?] We use our, we use the room. Or . . . I tend to use the private area to play and . . . yeah develop my relationship I guess with my baby um yeah, I've, I prefer to do that privately rather than publicly, I don't feel particularly comfortable developing that relationship in the communal room . . . But that's because I'm quite a private person.

Connie did not take advantage of the lounges and other shared areas to openly develop her relationship with her baby, it may have been a bit soon for her or perhaps, as she said, she was a more private person. A group of four women also discussed the limitations of Park House with respect to spaces they could connect with their babies and toddlers, or things which entertained the children:

Amelia: Well when there's little ones, you can usually put two on the mat but if he's [points to her child] in there, and he is a lot older, like you can put him with a baby but you've got to be careful because he's starting to move so I just, you know, worry, you know, [he might] fall over and fall on another baby so yeah.

Leah: Babies too and between their play time and their stomach time you really have to keep them separate but then you feel sorry for the older kids because it's really hard to move around and . . . you really only have your bedroom in the end.

Amelia: And that play area there [pointing to the play pen area] it's way too small.

Zara: It's very small . . . It's like a jail.

Leah: It's horrible I, I feel bad for my son when I lock him in there and then I come out here with my baby, um . . . the outdoor area is great but when the sun's out, no you get . . .

Overall, then, it seemed that the outside spaces were generally considered useful and enjoyable to be in, and fun for children. Participants particularly liked the opportunity to spend time in the sun and the playground spaces to keep older children entertained. Other participants also spoke about group therapy sessions happening outside and the beneficial aspects of spaces for such groups. However, service users felt that most other spaces in Park House weren't sufficiently well set up for their children—whether they were babies or toddlers.

SPACES FOR SLEEP AS LESS THAN IDEAL

Perhaps unsurprisingly, sleep was a key theme discussed by service users. As seen in previous themes, sleep issues included concerns about noise and light in rooms, which were frequently not seen as optimal by participants and which disrupted sleep for themselves and/or their children. Another example of this was provided in the following exchange between Amelia and Zara:

Amelia: I know with the nurseries sometimes, and I'm trying to put him to sleep it's like it's really noisy like when someone's opened the doors, or going to the bathroom or going to the cupboards it seems like . . . he is distracted very easily.

Zara: Very echoey.

Amelia: You've got the long hallway sort of thing between the nurseries and the other rooms that they use so I don't think they thought about that when they built the building like the nurseries shouldn't be

Zara: Yeah cos I'm trying to put him to sleep and the man's doing the linen and he's trying to be quiet obviously but he's just not and it's just like, you know, he won't settle.

Amelia: Yeah, the nurseries are right by the busiest area . . . Where all the traffic is.

Zara: And also, there is not much storage for everything so the nurseries are all cramped with stuff and sometimes it's really, really tight in there and you're trying to rock the cot to sleep and there's another cot there and another cot there and you're just like . . . really cramped.

Here, Zara and Amelia discuss a range of issues with the nurseries that caused problems with their babies' or toddlers' sleep—whether it be putting them to sleep in the first place (e.g., space issues when trying to rock them) or with things which woke them up (e.g., echoing noise). Other participants also mentioned issues with the available nurseries and cots, as seen in Beth's discussion with the interviewer below:

Beth: I think there needs to be more nurseries, honestly, there's only three and at the moment um my son and the other 18 month old that's here are both having to be in our rooms because there's not enough with the newborns which is fair enough but yeah it's a bit . . .

Interviewer: Not enough nurseries . . .

Beth: Yeah it gets a bit . . . Um . . . when I'm trying . . . I need to catch up on sleep as well and I might need time to myself and I can't really get that because he's *(sighs)*

Here, Beth discusses the need for more nurseries because her older toddler was having to sleep in the same room as her, which she indicated was disruptive for her own sleep. Beth also discussed the privacy impacts of having her toddler in her room with her, again highlighting the central role of privacy in participants' experiences of the space in Park House. Beth was not alone in this regard—many participants discussed the need for more nurseries, as seen in what Amelia says: "Yeah I think they need more nurseries 'cos, yeah, some nights, you know, babies are in the multi-purpose rooms and, or they have to be with you 'cos there's just no room."

Given that Park House was a purpose built MBU, it is curious that there were not enough nurseries within it to individually house at least one baby for every service user staying there (up to six at a time).

CONCLUDING THOUGHTS

Overall, participants were positive about much of the space at Park House. In particular, they appeared to like the sense of space, the light within the unit and the outdoor spaces. However, there were tensions in their relationship to the space and their expectations of it. This was particularly apparent in relation to the capacity for Park House to be "homely," while also recognizing that this was ultimately not a possibility given the functions that the space had to fulfill—namely that of safety, security, and elements of mental health care. As Tucker and colleagues (2019, 33) argue in relation to forensic mental health spaces: "A tension exists in terms of the capacities to create a home space in the ward, but to do so without the possibilities usually afforded by such spaces, e.g. privacy and personal control." Interestingly it was often participants who were not mothers (e.g., the two fathers and the mother-in-law who were interviewed) who discussed the importance of the space as encouraging mothers to interact with others in the unit and not spend time alone in bedrooms, perhaps suggesting discrepancies between what mothers wanted for themselves (privacy) and what those around them wanted in terms of the space.

Another element of service users' experiences was that the space did not seem to work well for relationship building with their children, or for their children to be entertained, a point we return to in chapter 7. Indeed, almost all service users felt that the space was better for babies or toddlers of a different age to their own. This mirrors discussions in chapter 3 regarding the limitations of the space for babies and toddlers, which is concerning given the design of the space as a mother–baby facility. Indeed, several of the mothers in particular were quite upset that there were no spaces they felt desirable/appropriate in which to connect with their children—drawing again on desires for privacy so as to work on mother–baby relationships. This was particularly the case for Connie, who had a very young baby (four weeks old), and who felt that there was nowhere she could go to get to know him, apart from her room, where she, her husband Geoff, and her mother-in-law all slept.

Indeed, sleep was another aspect of the space which service users felt was suboptimal. All participants reported problems with the sleep space (or the nursery space in general) to one degree or another, noting that the noise in particular (e.g., that of doors opening or closing, or hearing other babies or service users crying) either woke them directly or indirectly because it woke their baby. Given how important sleep is for well-being—particularly for new parents with small children (Montgomery-Downs, Stremler, and Insana 2013)—the fact that Park House was not well designed for promoting sleep seems problematic.

Chapter 7

Conclusion

In this final chapter of the book, we use the theme of "space" to explore the intersections of people and spaces in the context of both Park House and MBUs more broadly. In so doing, we take up some of the tensions evident in the analytic chapters of this book, tensions that are summarized well in the work of Fox (1999, 55), who suggests that "space is something which does not itself constrain, but which acts as a cue to ways of thinking about the world and the body." As he suggests, this means that "it is better to think about the built environment as offering *cues* to behavior" (Fox 1999, 50, emphasis in original). Certainly in some of the analytic chapters of this book, we have very much focused on the built space of Park House as an entity. Importantly, however, in taking this focus our purpose has not been to accord personhood to the built space. Rather, it has been to explore how the built space of Park House offers, in Fox's language, cues for thinking about how to act in the space. In this chapter, then, we explore how these cues may take multiple forms, focusing specifically on how the built space of Park House may serve to both regulate and dysregulate the people within it, how the space is peopled in diverse ways, and how the space offers cues for imagination that too are diverse.

Returning to some of the points we made in chapter 4, we also suggest that the built space of Park House provided cues for how we, as researchers, oriented ourselves. There were spaces in which we felt more comfortable (e.g., communal spaces such as the dining area), spaces where we felt observed (e.g., the garden area), and spaces upon which we felt at times we were intruding (e.g., the corridors near the bedrooms). Our feelings in these spaces were a product of our own subjectivities, the interactions we experienced with other people in Park House, and the cues given by the built space itself. We were aware that we were conducting research in a "sensitive" space, one that, for mothers potentially, was at times overpopulated by staff whose role was to monitor and observe. We were thus mindful that we potentially contributed to this sense of overpopulation and observation, and that we served as yet another cue in this regard. Further, our interactions with people in Park House were cued by our subjectivities as researchers, but they were also cued by our location as "known outsiders." Given the practices of observation outlined in chapter 4, and explored further below, our practices were in many ways out of step with the running of Park House: we sat still and watched, rather than moving around and interacting with mothers. Finally, we were very much cued by the space: which areas would offer us opportunities to observe (i.e., areas where there was high traffic); which areas spoke to our research interests. In being cued by the built space of Park House, its occupants, and our own subjectivities, then, we were thus cued to a particular reading of the space.

Our focus in this final chapter is therefore a situated discussion of space. As we saw in chapters 3, 5, and 6, other stakeholders had differing views on the built space of Park House, due to their own situatedness. Architects saw the space as a purpose built space, one that followed specific design principles, and which was deliberately intended to cue certain behaviors. Staff, in varying ways, saw the space as an inhabited space: inhabited by their own past experiences of the old MBU, inhabited by service users for whom they were responsible, and inhabited in ways that were the product of a space that was not always fit for purpose. Mothers generally saw the space as a welcoming space, one that could potentially facilitate well-being, but nonetheless a space with its own rules and regulations. There is, then, no one singular "space" of Park House. Rather, it is constituted by multiple spaces; each a product of individual imaginings, practices of habitation, needs, and past experiences. In many ways the built space of Park House allowed for these multiple readings of the space, while at the same time codifying particular cues about the space. It is to these cues that we now turn.

DYS/REGULATED SPACES

In this first section of the chapter we consider aspects of the built space of Park House, and MBUs more broadly, that speak to the idea that such units aim to regulate what is seen as dysregulation (i.e., poor mental health). In so doing, we also seek to consider how MBUs may, unintentionally, produce dysregulation, as a result of particular design features or approaches to care. Regulation and dysregulation, then, are two sides of the one coin in terms of the built space of MBUs, a claim that we feel is an important one to make in terms of having an expansive view of how these units as built spaces serve to produce particular cues in terms of their operations and functions.

Fraught Spaces

In many ways, Park House was a fraught space. It was fraught by design principles that did not always align with the needs of service users and staff, as we saw in chapters 4, 5, and 6. It was also fraught by the competing needs of observation, and the need to engender a homely space that could facilitate well-being. For us as researchers, it was fraught by a desire to blend in, or at least not be obtrusive as observers, but it was also fraught by our recognition of the fact that our location within the unit was in many ways very odd, and that we wanted people to be aware that we were there (especially if they did not consent to us monitoring their use of the space). Given the nature of the services provided by Park House, it was in many ways inevitable that it would be a fraught space. Here we want to explore, however, how the fraught nature of Park House sits within a continuum of such institutional spaces, with long and vexed histories.

As we outlined in chapter 1, we have very much seen a shift from the mental health institution as a highly medicalized and policed space to the creation of mental health institutions that aim to be welcoming, open, and homely. Yet, as Kaup (2011) notes in her research on aged care facilities, any shift in policy and practice is constrained by the space itself. Spaces, such as aged care homes or MBUs, may adopt an ethos of inclusion and openness, but this may not always be mirrored in the design of the built space. Some spaces remain marked as regulated, and all spaces remain spaces open to monitoring. Design features, including security cameras, nurses' stations, and the layout of rooms, may all too often retain the hallmarks of the historically more medicalized and policed space of the institution.

Moreover, and as Kaup (2011) has again argued, in spaces where domesticity and social labor collide, such as in aged care homes and MBUs, there is always a point of intersection where domesticity may serve to overlay or indeed mask the emotional labor involved. In MBUs specifically, the domestic features of such units, and the caring role that staff may play, potentially masks the regulatory aspects of the space. We explored this point briefly in chapter 4 and in more depth in chapter 6, but it is important to reiterate here that while we are mindful that regulation and domesticity must come hand in hand in MBUs, the question remains as to how their overlaps make the space itself a fraught space. If the space is one that emphasizes domesticity alongside clinical care, how can it be known in advance how service users will read the space? And how will service users' readings shape their engagement with services, and their awareness of the less-than-domestic aspects of the space?

In Park House specifically, mothers were provided with an introductory booklet, one that outlined the expectations and approaches adopted within Park House. What we don't know, however, is how mothers engaged with this material, particularly at the point of admission when they may have been in significant distress. While for mothers on mental health orders the question of consent may be somewhat moot, for mothers accommodated voluntarily the question about consent is imminently salient.

How to ensure that service users know what they are consenting to by being in the space of an MBU, and how, as is the case in other spheres, consent must be continually negotiated, is thus a question for the design and practice of future MBUs. It likely does not suffice to have one point of informational exchange, one point of drawing attention to features and practices within a unit. Rather, consent to observation, to regulation, and to treatment may well need to be continual: engendering conversations that remind mothers of their rights as well as obligations, and which frame staff as active participants in the space including in terms of regulation. To do otherwise is to reiterate a top-down model of power and control, which likely is at odds with the desired outcomes of MBUs (i.e., to support mothers to feel in control of their relationship with their child/ren).

Sensory Spaces

The space of Park House was very much a sensory space, though as we explored throughout this book, likely in ways that weren't necessarily intended. It was a "noisy" space, particularly in communal areas, as a result of the flooring and fixtures used. Shoes could be heard "clicking" on the floors. Doors could be heard shutting or slamming. Voices talking and phones ringing could be heard at some distance from the source of the sound, and often in ways that were discomforting: we could not always tell where particular sounds were coming from. Conversely, some aspects of the built space were positive from a sensory perspective. The bedroom wing allowed for the dampening of sounds and for the darkening of the space, so that mothers and babies could sleep, although the doors themselves created noise due to being heavy, meaning that they slammed shut (and needed to be muffled with hanging towels). The large windows in the dining area allowed for the warmth of the sunshine to enter the space in winter, although could also be blinding from the sun, and the outdoor areas were sensory in terms of the many textures used, the play equipment, and the landscaping. Park House, then, was a diverse space in terms of sensory outputs and inputs.

In the context of neonatal intensive care units, the importance of regulating sensory spaces has been increasingly recognized (White 2011). The temperature, smells, and lighting of the space impact not only on the child but also on their parents when visiting, as well as upon staff. In a similarly therapeutic space as an MBU, a focus on sensory inputs is thus likely equally important. Smells in particular can serve as a trigger for memories: both pleasant and unpleasant ones. When undertaking our observations in Park House, we noted that at some mealtimes the smell of what we perceived to be "packaged food" was often overwhelming, permeating the space. For some service users, this may be a familiar smell, evoking notions of home and mealtimes. For other service users, however, certain food-related smells may be triggers for less than pleasant memories, whether as a part of previous hospitalizations (including a potentially difficult birthing experience), or as part of growing up or adult life. Focus on the serving of food, and the smells generated, then, would seem an important part of attending to the sensory environment within MBUs.

Further in terms of sensory regulation, Park House did not include a seclusion space. This is likely because of the nature of the unit, which focused on mother–baby relationships. Women experiencing mental health concerns not amenable to focusing on the relationship would likely be housed in a generalist mental health unit. It is nonetheless notable to us that Park House did not include a specific space designated for sensory modulation. Certainly, as we noted above, the bedrooms could serve this function, as potentially darkened spaces where sounds were dampened. However, if a partner was staying with the mother, or if a baby was asleep in the room, of if the mother's distress was so significant as to potentially disrupt other people in the bedroom wing of Park House, it is salient that no specific space was designated where service users could go to take "time out" from potential sensory overload. Certainly, there were living room spaces and the outdoor areas, but these were not private. A service user could potentially sit in a consulting room, however even with locked filing cabinets these were not spaces conducive to having time out. For the future design of MBUs, then, the inclusion of a sensory time-out space may be a productive design feature that allows mothers (and potentially babies) a space to retreat from the noise and other forms of stimulation of the broader unit.

Developmentalist Spaces

Finally in terms of dys/regulation, we now consider how the space of Park House, and MBUs more broadly, orients to infants, and the types of orientation involved. In terms of the built space, Park House included a dedicated fenced off play space for small children, located alongside the dining area. This allowed small children to be in a secure area nearby to parents who may be eating. The play area included toys, as did the larger outside area, and toys and children's storybooks were also present in the main living area (located alongside the dining area). Yet beyond this, Park House was not clearly marked as a space designed for small children. Busy thoroughfares were not areas that small children, and especially toddlers, could play. The dining area was an open area adjoining a walkway, and while there were ample highchairs available, a child walking around while a parent ate could potentially be at risk due to people passing through the area. While the garden areas were pleasantly landscaped, the presence of plants and flowers were not without risk to small children; additionally due to occupational health and safety requirements the external doors could not be left open for children to move easily between spaces. Thinking developmentally, then, in terms of the needs and interests of small children, Park House was not necessarily a space built for them.

In terms of development more broadly, Park House, like other MBUs, focused its therapeutic efforts on attachment. As Burman (2007, 130) has argued, attachment is the "trope, lynchpin or turning point around which mothers [are] evaluated and regulated." Indeed, for many mothers housed in Park House and other MBUs, attachment is seen as a problem to be corrected. In her study of an MBU, Masciantonio (2015) notes that theories about attachment serve as justification for the admission of women. Problems with attachment become the logic by which admission and discharge are determined, following a relatively narrow script about what constitutes a positive attachment relationship. Arguably, as Masciantonio suggests, the attachment focus of MBUs very much serves to ensure a focus on children. But, at the same time, it serves to ensure a focus on the attachment models of service users, potentially problematizing their own upbringing and experiences of attachment, and viewing these as requiring "work" in order to resolve potential attachment issues in the present.

While not without its utility, attachment theory, then, as a central principal of MBUs, serves to enshrine a highly normative view of mother-baby relationships. It is developmentalist in that it provides a lens through which to evaluate mothers and babies. It is developmentalist in the sense that it postulates one idealized outcome for attachment (a secure attachment). And it is developmentalist in that it suggests that it is professionals who can diagnose and treat attachment issues. Certainly, MBUs require an organizing logic through which to facilitate treatment. But the question here remains as to the degree to which the logic of attachment theory shapes the built space itself. MBUs provide hands-on assistance by staff to help facilitate the "repair" of attachment relationships. But, as was the case for Park House, the design of the space may not readily be viewed as legible in terms of attachment. As we outlined in chapter 4, Park House included somewhat fragmented spaces that were at times are a simulacrum of home, but were never actually home. Similarly, the regulation of spaces open to service users, such as the client kitchen from which children were prohibited, potentially maintained safety as much as they served as cues *against* or *unsupportive of* attachment needs. While we did not specifically ask service users or staff about how the built space facilitated attachment, it will be important into the future that purpose built designs investigate how spaces do or do not speak to a focus on attachment, and whether or not they provide cues to an attachment focus.

PEOPLED SPACES

In the first section above we focused on how the built space of MBUs, including Park House, are spaces that are both highly regulated, but which may nonetheless produce dysregulation. This is because such spaces are fraught by tensions between being healthy environments and regulatory environments, due to such spaces being "noisy," and because such spaces rely upon developmentalist assumptions. In this next section we shift to explore how the built spaces of MBUs are peopled: peopled by staff, by mothers, and by visitors. As peopled spaces, MBUs potentially draw attention to normative understandings of subjectivity, specifically with regard to gender, sexuality, class, and culture. It is to these aspects of subjectivity that we now turn to examine.

Gendered Spaces

In her classic text *Space, Place and Gender*, Massey (1994, 186) writes that the "gendering of space and place both reflects *and has effects back on* the ways in which gender is constructed and understood in the societies in which we live" (emphasis in original). In the context of MBUs, it is perhaps understandable that the built space gives gendered cues, given the primary focus on people of one particular gender (i.e., women). Yet, as we noted in the previous section on developmentalism, and following Massey, we might argue that developmentalist spaces have effects back on women, specifically regarding constructions of, and judgments about, women who are mothers. Further in terms of the built space and women, and as we touched on in chapters 1, 3, and 4 and will explore more in the section below, the domesticity inherent to MBUs normatively marks the space as specifically gendered, given the long-standing normative associations between women, mothering, and carework. In other words, the very fact that "mother-baby units" exist (i.e., not "parent-baby units"), and the fact that such units increasingly seek to replicate to a certain degree the family home, tells us much about how the space gives cues to gender that are normative. Furthermore, and as we noted in chapter 3, given that the space of Park House was designed primarily by men who are architects, it is perhaps not surprising that an "outsiders" view of what constitutes a domestic (and thus by default maternal) space would be evoked.

Importantly, however, MBUs are not simply gendered by the fact that they focus primarily on women. They are also gendered by the provision they make (or not) for people of other genders to occupy the space. In Park House, for example, we noted in our ethnographic observations that one male nurse worked in the unit, and we often heard comment that he was a useful resource for fathers visiting the unit. This was especially the case with regard to regular barbeques that were held when family members were visiting, and where the male staff member was seen as an important conduit to engage male visitors in the context of preparing food. This type of gendered practice evokes normative assumptions about men wanting to speak to other men, thus potentially marginalizing the voices of the primarily female staff and service users. Indeed, we might suggest that the assumption that men will primarily want to talk to other men is part of the problem in terms of heterosexual couples where mothers experience postpartum mental health concerns, and the felt need to turn to people outside of their partner for support.

Having suggested that potentially part of the problem facing mothers experiencing postpartum mental health concerns are normative assumptions about gender, it is nonetheless important to acknowledge that for men, such concerns experienced by female partners can be challenging. Research by Boddy and colleagues (2017), for example, has found that men are often unaware that a female partner may face challenges postpartum, with hospitalization often occurring quite quickly, leaving men unsure about what lies ahead, and feeling disengaged from health services. In Boddy et al.'s (2017) research, for men who felt excluded from the information exchange in the context of hospitalization due to postpartum mental health concerns, anger was a common response. This response, potentially exacerbating the types of gender divides that we suggested above, may be part of the problem. Men were often left to feel as though they were "holding the fort," many of whom had little experience in running the household or caring for older children, again due to normative gendered practices and assumptions.

In her MBU study, Masciantonio (2015) noted that at times fathers were permitted to stay with mothers in the unit, though only if the staff determined that this was in the best interest of the mother, the mother–child relationship, and the other service users. In part the logic behind this approach related to the fact that, for some women, admission to the unit may have involved a history of having experienced domestic violence from a male partner, and that having a man stay in the unit could be problematic. At the same time, however, and as was the case for Park House, in addition to the single male nurse, at least three male staff members responsible for the garden, laundry, and security worked in/frequented the unit, and there were often male visitors. The assumption that quarantining men off as "boarders," then, has to be located in the broader context of a unit that was *not* a woman-only space. Different to a domestic violence unit, then, MBUs are mixed gender spaces, and it is possible that in an effort to focus on safety from women, broader normative assumptions about gendered interactions were being reiterated in the space of the MBU. Specifically, keeping fathers often at an arm's length meant that the normative expectation that mothers provide primary care for children was reiterated. Undoubtedly the father's own mental health is a crucial component in MBUs (Reid et al. 2017), and our data show that one father was admitted soon after the mother at Park House. Nonetheless, a whole-of-family approach appeared to be encouraged at Park House and in line with others (Grube 2005; Kemp 2011; Turner, Garrett, and Wittkowski 2018) it is likely that length of stay can be reduced for women with supportive partnerships.

Diverse Spaces

Importantly, MBUs such as Park House are not only marked by gender differences. They are also marked by diversity in culture, sexuality, and class. In chapter 4 we explored briefly how some of the design and practice features of Park House potentially relied upon particular classed assumptions about what mothers would want from the space (e.g., a television always being on). As a public service, but as the only such service in the state, Park House notionally serviced all mothers who required mental health care with their small children. Yet we might suggest, and potentially reflecting the specific service users seen by staff, that the space was in fact tailored toward a very specific, class-based view of a particular cohort of clientele. It will certainly be important for future research to examine more closely how class-based assumptions shape the design and practice of MBUs, including in how staff position themselves in the context of class, and how this intersects with the lives of the mothers they work with.

Further in terms of diversity, Park House and likely other MBUs are not restricted to the housing of heterosexual mothers and their infants. During our ethnographic observations, for example, we saw one mother housed in the unit visited by her female partner. In terms of our observations this was a challenge, as while we were mindful of heteronormativity, it was somewhat easier to "read" a male visitor as the partner of a woman housed in the unit (though this was not always the case), while female visitors could be friends, sisters, and mothers. This speaks again to normative gendered practices, where it was less likely that male friends, brothers, or fathers would visit women staying in Park House, meaning that male visitors were more readily identifiable as likely to be partners and/or fathers. In the case of the female partner visitor, it took a number of visits for us to determine that she was the partner of the mother she was visiting. The visibility of women with women partners in MBUs is salient, given that research suggests that such women experience postpartum mental health concerns on par with heterosexual women, yet may experience fear in seeking help due to concerns that others would judge them as lesbian mothers, and that as a result their children might be taken away from them (Alang and Fomotar 2015). This highlights the importance of considering how MBUs potentially speak to or simply repeat normative assumptions about gender as much as they speak to or simply repeat normative assumptions about sexuality. This includes in the language used in information packs, in promotional information about the unit, in group sessions, and in other situations where gender and sexuality may be normatively marked.

Another aspect of diversity, and one that we covered to some extent in chapter 3, pertains to cultural sensitivity and diversity. During our ethnographic observations there was little diversity in the cultural backgrounds of women in the unit. Our interviews with staff, however, certainly oriented at times to the topic of the inclusion of women from diverse cultural backgrounds. This is important, given research suggests that migrant and refugee women may be especially vulnerable to postpartum depression (O'Mahony et al. 2013). For some women of diverse cultural backgrounds, mental health may be a taboo topic within families, encouraging silence about the challenges that they face after the birth of a child. Some women of diverse cultural backgrounds, however, may find avenues to support through religious practices, which may be viewed as a positive strength in terms of coping with postpartum mental health concerns. It is of note, then, that Park House did not provide an all faith prayer space. Certainly, women and visitors could use spaces such as bedrooms in which to pray, but these are not ideal spaces for worship. That the built space of Park House did not speak to the needs of women of diverse cultural backgrounds, for some of whom religion may be an important part of their cultural practice, thus is telling with regard to the design of the space being mindful (or not) of cultural diversity and its impact on maternal well-being.

Masciantonio (2015) further notes, from her study of an MBU, that such units typically endorse highly culturally normative ideals about sleeping (e.g., no co-sleeping), mealtime, and sleep time. As Masciantonio notes, such ideals, when evident in MBUs, while potentially meeting the needs of culturally dominant group members whose beliefs and practices may align with those considered appropriate in terms of eating and sleeping, may nonetheless fail to meet the needs of women from other cultural groups. Furthermore, and as we explored in the section above on developmentalism, in Park House specifically attachment theory was a key organizing principle. The cultural specificity of attachment theory as a belief system was not something that appeared to be recognized in Park House, meaning that women of diverse cultural backgrounds might well be subjected to a belief system about parenting that was out of step with their own cultural practices (Keller 2016). This suggests the importance of not only MBUs recognizing a diversity of cultural practices when it comes to sleeping, meals, and "attachment," but also the potential need for therapeutic spaces for mothers and their children that are specifically directed toward women of diverse cultural backgrounds.

Finally in terms of diversity, we note that although Park House encouraged visits from family members, and was able to accommodate partners of mothers in some instances, the unit policy did not permit nonhuman animals to visit the facility. While, as we learnt from conversations with staff, in some cases exceptions could be made to this policy, exceptions were typically made with regard to smaller animals, and was contingent on whether or not toddlers were present in the unit (which stemmed from concerns about the risk of larger animals—such as dogs—to toddlers). Given the central role of animal companions in the family lives of many people (Charles and Davies 2011), and given the role that such companions can play in facilitating positive mental health outcomes (Brooks et al. 2018), it is thus notable that they are largely excluded from the facility. Fox and Ray (2019), in their research on aged care facilities, have also found that animals are often excluded, and have suggested that this can be a significant source of grief for older humans separated from animals when they enter into an aged care home. Whether or not women admitted to MBUs similarly experience grief upon separation from animals (among other family members) is a topic for further research.

Importantly in regards to animals in the space of MBUs, however, we must raise the question of what it means for small animals (such as hamsters) to visit such units, given such animals have physical frames that are likely delicate, and are thus at risk of harm when handled by multiple people. How the space of Park House, along with other MBUs, makes possible nonhuman visitors, and indeed how it could potentially incorporate animals into its therapeutic approach, is most certainly a matter for continued examination; however, this requires attention to the implications of visits for animals who may find the space strange, who may be at risk of unintended harm (including during travel) and who may themselves experience separation distress when brought for a visit only to be taken away again.

IMAGINED SPACES

In the previous section we focused on how MBUs, such as Park House, are variously peopled, and we emphasized the importance of focusing on the diversity of people who may interact with the built space. This section builds on the previous section by considering how the built space of Park House, like other MBUs, is an imagined space. As we noted in chapter 3, Park House is an imagined space in the context of its location on grounds that previously housed psychiatric facilities based on ideas from a previous century. As such, it constitutes part of a trajectory of a more traditional facility: it is not entirely free of that history. As such even within the new, purpose built, space, Park House evokes imaginaries that are not entirely determined by the design. Certainly, as we noted in the introduction to this chapter, the built space gives cues to particular imaginaries, but it is not entirely limited to them. We take up this point by first examining the potentially homely nature of the built space, a more familiar and common imaginary. We then turn to contrast this with the idea of Park House, and other MBUs, as a temporary or transitional space, eliciting its own forms of imaginary.

Homely Spaces

As we documented in chapters 3, 4, 5, and 6, certain aspects of the design of Park House mark it as a homely space. From the spaces that may mark it as home (e.g., bedrooms, living areas, kitchens), to the design features (e.g., children's toys, clotheslines), Park House cues its inhabitants to read it as home. Yet as [Author] (2019) notes in her examination of an aged care facility, spaces that are cued to be seen as home can be "ruptured." Movement into an MBU specifically brings with it a removal from a homely space, into a space that presents a simulacrum of home, but is purposively *not* a home. The question that remains, then, and one that [Author] asks, is how, as a simulation of home, built spaces such as aged care facilities or MBUs potentially paper over the ruptures produced by the differences between one's home, and the semblance of home created in such spaces.

As [Author] (2019) notes, part of our focus, then when it comes to the built space of MBUs, is the communication that occurs between the space and its occupants. Just as the built space of an MBU may serve as a cue for home, we must understand how service users and staff take up or refuse such cues. In our observations, for example, we noted that mothers, and at times visitors, wore pyjamas, or slippers, or socks or other items of clothing that gave a sense of being "at home." Yet at the same time, such clothing might be worn in a hospital, thus suggesting that the cues offered by the space were potentially multiple: mothers were both home and away. Similarly, as might also be the case at home, mothers and visitors at times appeared to enjoy "lounging" in the place, suggesting that the space achieved in its capacity to provide cues to a convivial space in which people could linger. Yet at the same time, sometimes mothers and visitors appeared less than comfortable in the space, such as when they ate meals in the dining area and then left for their bedroom (which, to follow up a point raised earlier in this chapter, may have been a product of our presence: they may have wished to avoid further observation). This might speak to individual mental health concerns, or a desire for privacy, but it might also speak to the limits to which the space was felt to be home.

Another aspect of the space that was potentially homely was the capacity for mothers to prepare meals for themselves or their children, and the encouragements to take care of the space in terms of cleaning. Other than the signs in the "client kitchen," these were all things people might do at home (i.e., cook and clean). Importantly, however, the space of Park House was staffed by cleaners, who took care of much of the cleaning work. The presence of cleaners, while an important occupational health and safety feature of MBUs, is a cue that the space is not home, but rather a space that approximates home. This is especially the case given that while some mothers in MBUs may employ people to clean their houses, in the MBU itself someone else is doing the employing, and thus someone else is giving the directives to clean. Interestingly, we noted that some mothers potentially sought to bridge this divide by developing their own relationships with cleaning staff, thus potentially bringing them into their own fold, or bridging the divide between them as cleaning staff and service users. Either way, and given we did not interview cleaning staff, future research would greatly benefit from surveying the views of cleaning staff, and their role in MBUs.

In their own work on aged care facilities, Kaup (2011) suggests that doors serve a particular function in terms of regulating the public/private divide, and in terms of creating a semblance of home. As we noted in chapters 3, 4, 5, and 6, some doors were accessible only to staff, some doors were not fit for purpose (e.g., bedroom or nursery doors that closed too loudly), and some doors gave a modicum of privacy, but that privacy was not absolute (e.g., bedroom doors could be opened by staff). Kaup (2011) suggests that attention to doors and their capacity to manage the space between private and public are an important design feature that requires attention in terms of evoking a sense of home. Certainly, in an MBU, lockable doors in spaces accessible to service users must be limited, given that some service users may experience considerable distress. Yet at the same time, we need to ask how service users view the functions of doors: do they screen out, or lock in, or lock out, or fulfill some other criterion that may facilitate or reduce the likelihood that the space will be considered to be homelike. As Kaup (2011) notes, doors, as but one design feature, cue inhabitants to the space. How doors cue the inhabitants of MBUs is thus an important topic for future research.

Temporary Spaces

Contrary to MBUs being a homely space, it is also a temporary space. While admission periods are not fixed (with one mother being in Park House for the duration of our observations), they are intended to serve as a temporary solution that produces outcomes that translate into more sustainable solutions (i.e., returning home, even if that requires ongoing outpatient support). Indeed, this tension between the homely and the temporary may speak to why the built space of Park House was ultimately, in our reading, not an entirely homely space. It could not be entirely homely because it was not home. It could not be entirely homely because it needed to meet occupational health and safety standards not typically required in homes. But importantly, it was not intended to be a permanent home.

How, then, do MBUs such as Park House speak to the homely and the temporary? Masciantonio (2015), in her ethnography of an MBU, suggests that this binary of home and transition is managed in MBUs by a dual focus on creating a caring environment, but one that is always directed toward a return home. Mothers may need to fulfill certain requirements, or meet certain goals, before they can return home. The space, then, while in terms of design being somewhat homely, is ultimately framed therapeutically as a transitional space. Indeed, we might liken the MBU to Winnicott's (1953) concept of the transitional object. A transitional object for a child, such as a blanket or toy, can help children move between spaces, compensating for change. The built space of the MBU, then, might serve as a transitional space. It is homely enough to not be entirely strange, but at the same time it is not home because it serves a purpose not possible at home. This would suggest, then, that research on how MBUs function as, or are understood as, transitional spaces is vital.

Importantly, in terms of MBUs as transitional or temporary spaces, we must also be mindful that they are potentially such spaces not only for mothers but also for staff. Staff working in MBUs spend a considerable portion of their working hours in the unit, yet it is a space designed to appear like home. Certainly, the staff wing of Park House was much more like a regular office, however it overlooked the larger garden area (via an internal walkway), and staff did not spend all of their time in this wing. The nurses' station, by comparison, was located in between the communal areas of the unit and the bedroom wing. While notionally situated for observation, it also was situated as part of the "home" of the unit. Our point here is not to question whether or not staff could distinguish between work and home. Rather, it is to raise a query as to how the homely aspects of the unit were potentially at cognitive odds with the work that staff were doing as professionals. Staff moved in and out of Park House as their workplace, but in so doing they moved from a home to homelike space, but with the latter requiring particular attention to regulations and therapeutic work. How all staff, and not just clinical staff, understand this divide, then, will be an important topic for future research.

HEALTHY SPACES

Having considered in the previous section some of the imaginaries at play in MBUs that are at once both home and away (or temporary or transitional), in this final section we consider how such spaces are healthy spaces. In chapter 1 we outlined extensively the remit of architecture and design for well-being. As such, we do not wish to simply repeat this discussion here. Rather, our query relates to the degree to which built spaces, and MBUs specifically, can ever truly be healthy spaces. Certainly as we have seen in the chapters in this book, certain design features, and practice principles, orient to the aim of well-being. As such, Park House meets its brief. Yet, we would be remiss if we limited our discussion to the positive or negative effects of the design itself. As we noted in the introduction to this chapter, the design of a space gives cues: it does not predetermine readings of those cues.

With the above point about cues and readings in mind, we suggest here that design for health is but one part of healthy spaces. Equally, if not more important, are the relationships that occur within built spaces. Certainly, some spaces may cue or facilitate positive relationships more than do other spaces, but at their core spaces must cue relationships. In MBUs, these are relationships between mothers and their babies, between mothers and their families, between mothers and their own self-understandings, all facilitated through relationships between staff and service users. This leads us to suggest that there is no one definitively "healthy space." A space can be a conduit to well-being through its design, but if it is not a conduit to relationships, it will likely fail. In Park House, certain aspects of the design were conduits to relationships (e.g., communal areas, a nurses' station that could be accessed by service users), though others were potentially less conducive (e.g., aspects of regulation, the structure of the outdoor areas). This meant, then, that at times staff were potentially working with and against the design of the space to facilitate relationships with service users (and indeed with one another).

We might suggest, then, that "design for health" is more correctly "design that isn't counter to healthy relationships." Certainly in this book and in our other work, we have identified plenty of examples of what would *not* constitute design for health in the context of mental health units (Authors 2015). By contrast, in many ways in this book we have focused on design and practice principles that are not counter to healthy relationships. In so doing, we have identified barriers to healthy relationships (e.g., who can visit, how diversity is understood), facilitators of health relationships (e.g., accessible and welcoming spaces that enable positive relationships), and we have also suggested areas where more work is yet to be done on what might constitute spaces that facilitate healthy relationships in the context of MBUs.

CONCLUDING THOUGHTS

Taking up the points raised at the end of the previous section, we would suggest in conclusion to this book that we have opened up new vistas for thinking about "design for health" in MBUs. We have endorsed aspects of the design and practice of Park House, just as much as we have explored its limitations. In so doing, we have questioned what it means for a space to be "purpose built," suggesting that any such build must truly understand and appreciate its purpose. In this book we have further honed, from a design and post occupancy evaluation perspective, where Park House adhered to its stated purpose by its design, and where it might have done better. We have done this by drawing on our own observations, and the views of architects, staff, and service users. This, we believe, gives a holistic view of the design of Park House, and speaks more broadly to the design of MBUs.

In conclusion, this book holds in tension many aspects of the built space and use of MBUs. These are tensions that relate to observation and therapeutic agendas, being at home and being in a temporary or transitional space, being comfortable and following regulations, being welcoming and following protocols, and being broadly inclusive while focusing on a specific group of people (i.e., mothers). Our goal in writing this book was never to resolve these tensions: they are inherent to MBUs. Nonetheless, our goal was very much to draw attention to these tensions, and by so doing opening up opportunities for new ways of thinking about the design and use of MBUs. As spaces that are both home and away, MBUs will always be required to negotiate with tensions, but ideally this should be to the benefit and with the consent and understanding of all who occupy the space.

Bibliography

Abel, Kathryn M., Roger T. Webb, Margaret P. Salmon, Ming W. Wan, and Louis Appleby. 2005. "Prevalence and Predictors of Parenting Outcomes in a Cohort of Mothers with Schizophrenia Admitted for Joint Mother and Baby Psychiatric Care in England." *The Journal of Clinical Psychiatry* 66 (6): 781–789.

Adams, Laurie Schneider. 2005. *A History of Western Art*. Boston: McGraw Hill.

Agrest, Diane. 2000. "Architecture from Without: Body, Logic and Sex." In *Gender, Space, Architecture: An Interdisciplinary Introduction*, edited by Jane Rendell, Barbara Penner, and Iain Borden, 358–370. London: Routledge.

Alang, S. M., and Fomotar, M. 2015. "Postpartum Depression in an Online Community of Lesbian Mothers: Implications for Clinical Practice." *Journal of Gay & Lesbian Mental Health* 19 (1): 21–39.

Andes, Melanie, and Mona M. Shattell. 2006. "An Exploration of the Meaning of Space and Place in Acute Psychiatric Care." *Issues in Mental Health Nursing* 27 (6): 699–707.

Anjali, Joseph, Herminia Machry, Zahra Zamani, and Robert Davis. "Impact of Light on Outcomes in Healthcare Settings – A Review", paper presented at *Innovation: Shifting Ground*, Raleigh Convention Centre, Raleigh, North Carolina, 20 May 2016.

Antonysamy, Arokia, Angelika Wieck, and Anja Wittkowski. 2009. "Service Satisfaction on Discharge from a Psychiatric Mother and Baby Unit: A Representative Patient Survey." *Archives of Women's Mental Health* 12 (5): 359–362.

Archer, Michaela, Yasmine Lau, and Faisil Sethi. 2016. "Women in Acute Psychiatric Units, Their Characteristics and Needs: A Review." *BJPsych Bulletin* 40 (5): 266–272.

Baker, A., Mary Morison, J. A. Game, and J. G. Thorpe. 1961. "Admitting Schizophrenic Mothers with Their Babies." *Lancet* 278 (7196): 237–239.

Bartlett, Annie, and Nadia Somers. 2017. "Are Women Really Difficult? Challenges and Solutions in the Care of Women in Secure Services." *The Journal of Forensic Psychiatry & Psychology* 28 (2): 226–241.

Bauer, Annette, Michael Parsonage, Martin Knapp, Valentina Iemmi, and Bayo Adelaja. 2014. *The Costs of Perinatal Mental Health Problems.* London: Centre for Mental Health and London School of Economics.

Biancheri, Rita, and Stefania Landi. 2016. "Health, Gender and Health-Care Design: Considerations About Hospital Environments in a Gender-Sensitive Perspective." *Italian Gender Specific Medicine* 2 (4): 158–160.

Bilszta, Justin L. C., Anne E. Buist, Fandy Wang, and Nur Rusydina Zulkefli. 2012. "Use of Video Feedback Intervention in an Inpatient Perinatal Psychiatric Setting to Improve Maternal Parenting." *Archives of Women's Mental Health* 15 (4): 249–257.

Boddy, Rebecca, Carolyn Gordon, Fiona MacCallum, and Mary McGuinness. 2017. "Men's Experiences of Having a Partner Who Requires Mother and Baby Unit Admission for First Episode Postpartum Psychosis." *Journal of Advanced Nursing* 73 (2): 399–409.

Bowlby, John. 1969. *Attachment and Loss: Vol. 1. Attachment.* New York: Basic Books.

Boyer, Kate. 2018. *Spaces and Places of Motherhood.* London: Rowan & Littlefield.

Braun, Virginia, and Victoria Clarke. 2006. "Using Thematic Analysis in Psychology." *Qualitative Research in Psychology* 3 (2): 77–101.

Breggin, Peter. 1991. *Toxic Psychiatry.* New York: St Martins Press.

Brockington, Ian, Ruth Butterworth, and Nine Glangeaud-Freudenthal. 2017. "An International Position Paper on Mother-Infant (Perinatal) Mental Health, with Guidelines for Clinical Practice." *Archives of Women's Mental Health* 20 (1): 113–120.

Brooks, Helen Louise, Kelly Rushton, Karina Lovell, Penny Bee, Lauren Walker, Laura Grant, and Anne Rogers. 2018. "The Power of Support from Companion Animals for People Living with Mental Health Problems: A Systematic Review and Narrative Synthesis of the Evidence." *BMC Psychiatry* 18 (1): 31.

Bryon, Els, Bernadette Dierckx de Casterlé, Chris Gastmans, Els Steeman, and Koen Milisen. 2008. "Mealtime Care on a Geriatric-Psychiatric Ward from the Perspective of the Caregivers: A Qualitative Case Study Design." *Issues in Mental Health Nursing* 29 (5): 471–494.

Buist, Anne, Bruno Minto, Klara Szego, M. Samhuel, L. Shawyer, and Lisa G. O'Connor. 2004. "Mother-Baby Psychiatric Units in Australia – The Victorian Experience." *Archives of Women's Mental Health* 7 (1): 81–87.

Buist, Anne E., Lorraine Dennerstein, and Graham D. Burrows. 1990. "Review of a Mother-Baby Unit in a Psychiatric Hospital." *Australian and New Zealand Journal of Psychiatry* 24 (1): 103–108.

Burman, Erica. 2007. *Deconstructing Developmental Psychology* (2nd Edition). New York: Routledge.

Butler, Hannah. 2013. "Parenting Interventions on a Mother and Baby Unit: An Investigation." Doctor of Clinical Psychology diss., The University of Manchester.

Butler, Hannah, Dougal Hare, Samantha Walker, Angelika Wieck, and Anja Wittkowski. 2014. "The Acceptability and Feasibility of the Baby Triple P

Positive Parenting Programme on a Mother and Baby Unit: Q-Methodology with Mothers with Severe Mental Illness." *Archives of Women's Mental Health* 17 (5): 455–463.

Butler, Judith. 1993. *Bodies That Matter: On the Discursive Limits of 'Sex'*. London: Routledge.

Butler, Judith. 2004. *Precarious Life: The Powers of Mourning and Violence.* London: Verso.

Butler-Coyne, Hannah, Dougal Hare, Samantha Walker, Angelika Wieck, and Anja Wittkowski. 2017. "Acceptability of a Positive Parenting Programme on a Mother and Baby Unit: Q-Methodology with Staff." *Journal of Child and Family Studies* 26 (2): 623–632.

Cantwell, Roch. 2016. "Maternal Perinatal Psychopathology: Overview." In *Joint Care of Parents and Infants in Perinatal Psychiatry*, edited by Anne-Laure Sutter-Dallay, Nine M-C Glangeaud-Freudenthal, Antoine Guedeney, and Anita Riecher-Rössler, 13–24. Cham: Springer.

Cazas, Odile, and Nine M.-C. Glangeaud-Freudenthal. 2004. "The History of Mother-Baby Units (MBUs) in France and Belgium and of the French Version of the Marcé Checklist." *Archives of Women's Mental Health* 7 (1): 53–58.

Cès, Agathe, Bruno Falissard, Nine M. C. Glangeaud-Freudenthal, Anne-Laure Sutter-Dallay, and Florence Gressier. 2018. "Pregnancy in Women with Psychotic Disorders: Risk Factors associated with Mother-Baby Separation." *Archives of Women's Mental Health* 21 (6): 699–706.

Chandra, Prabha S., Geetha Desai, Dharma Reddy, Harish Thippeswamy, and Gayatri Saraf. 2015. "The Establishment of a Mother-Baby Inpatient Psychiatry Unit in India: Adaptation of a Western Model to Meet Local Cultural and Resource Needs." *Indian Journal of Psychiatry* 57 (3): 290–294.

Charles, Nickie, and Charlotte Aull Davies. 2011. "My Family and Other Animals: Pets As Kin." In *Human and Other Animals: Critical Perspectives*, edited by Bob Carter and Nickie Charles, 69–92. London: Palgrave Macmillan.

Chodorow, Nancy Julia. 2012. *Gender and Sexuality: Theory and Practice.* London: Routledge.

Chousein, Berrin Chatzi. 2015. "Henning Larsen Architects Wins Competition of New Mental Health Building at Bispebjerg Hospital." *Turkey Architecture News*, May 28, 2015.

Christl, Bettina, Nicole Reilly, Carolyn Yin, and Marie-Paule Austin. 2015. "Clinical Profile and Outcomes of Women Admitted to a Psychiatric Mother-Baby Unit." *Archives of Women's Mental Health* 18 (6): 805–816.

Chrysikou, Evangelia. 2014. *Architecture for Psychiatric Environments and Therapeutic Spaces.* Amsterdam: IOS Press.

Clarke, Victoria, and V. Virginia Braun. 2013. *Successful Qualitative Research: A Practical Guide for Beginners*. London: Sage.

Connellan, Kathleen. 2010a. "White and Fitted: Perpetuating Modernisms." *Journal of Design Issues* 26 (3): 51–62.

Connellan, Kathleen. 2010b. "At Home: A Discussion of Diaspora and Hybridity." In *Interior Spaces in Other Places: IDEA (Interior Design Architecture Educators*

Association) Symposium, edited by Mark Taylor, Gini Lee, and Marissa Lindqiust. Brisbane: Queensland University of Technology. https://idea-edu.com/symposiums/2010-interior-space-in-other-places/

Connellan, Kathleen. 2016. "The Cult of Domesticity." In *The Wiley-Blackwell Encyclopedia of Gender and Sexuality Studies*, edited by Nancy Naples, Renee C. Hoogland, Maithree Wickramasinghe, and Wai Ching Angela Wong. Maryland, MD, United States: Wiley-Blackwell.

Connellan, Kathleen. 2018. "My Room, My Home, My Self." *Home Cultures* 15 (2): 103–127.

Connellan, Kathleen, Clare Bartholomaeus, Clemence Due, and Damien W. Riggs. 2017. "A Systematic Review of Research on Psychiatric Mother Baby Units." *Archives of Women's' Mental Health (AWMH)* 20: 373–388.

Connellan, Kathleen, Clemence Due, and Damien W. Riggs. 2015. "Light Lies: How Glass Speaks." *Communication Design Quarterly* 3 (4): 14–24.

Connellan, Kathleen, Mads Gaardboe, Damien W. Riggs, Clemence Due, Amanda Reinschmidt, and Lauren Mustillo. 2013. "Stressed Spaces: Mental Health and Architecture, A Review of the Literature." *Health Environments Research and Design Journal (HERD)* 6 (4): 127–168.

Connellan, Kathleen Anne. 2019. *Dreaming, Healing and Imaginative Arts Practice*. London: Routledge-Taylor Francis.

Connerty, Tracy Jayne, Rachel Roberts, and Anne Sved Williams. 2016. "Managing Life, Motherhood and Mental Health after Discharge from a Mother–Baby Unit: An Interpretive Phenomenological Analysis." *Community Mental Health Journal* 52 (8): 954–963.

Cooper, David. 2001. *Psychiatry and Anti-Psychiatry*. Oxford: Routledge.

Copperman, Jeannette, and Karen Knowles. 2006. "Developing Women Only and Gender Sensitive Practices in Inpatient Wards – Current Issues and Challenges." *The Journal of Adult Protection* 8 (2): 20–24.

Crocker, Catherine. 2013–2014. "Piloting of a National Perinatal Patient Satisfaction Scale – Feedback and Patient Satisfaction in Perinatal Mental Health Services." BMedSc Project Report, University of Southampton. https://www.rcpsych.ac.uk/pdf/CatherineCrocker.pdf

Crossley, Michele. 2000. *Rethinking Health Psychology*. Buckingham, Philadelphia: Open University Press.

Daniels, Yolande J. 2000. "Black Bodies, Black Space: A Waiting Spectacle." In *White Papers Black Marks: Architecture, Race, Culture*, edited by Lesly Naa Norle Lokko, 194–217. Minneapolis: University of Minnesota Press.

Deleuze, Gilles. 1992. "What Is a Dispositif?" In *Michel Foucault Philosopher: Essays Translated for the French and German*, edited by Timothy J. Armstrong, 159–168. New York: Routledge.

Douglas, Gwen. 1956. "Psychotic Mothers." *The Lancet* 267 (6908): 124–125.

Due, Clemence, Kathleen Connellan, and Damien W. Riggs. 2012. "Surveillance, Security and Violence in a Mental Health Ward: An Ethnographic Study of an Australian Purpose-Built Unit." *Surveillance and Society* 10 (3/4): 292–302.

Edwards, Clive. 2011. *Interior Design: A Critical Introduction*. Oxford: Berg.

Elkin, Amanda, Helen Gilburt, Mike Slade, Brynmor Lloyd-Evans, Alain Gregoire, Sonia Johnson, and Louise M. Howard. 2009. "A National Survey of Psychiatric Mother and Baby Units in England." *Psychiatric Services* 60 (5): 629–633.

Ferguson, Monika, James Dollman, Martin Jones, Kathryn Cronin, Lynne James, Lee Martinez, and Nicholas Procter. 2019. "Suicide Prevention Training–Improving the Attitudes and Confidence of Rural Australian Health and Human Service Professionals." *Crisis* 40 (1): 15–26.

Forty, Adrian. 1984. "The Modern Hospital in England and France: The Social and Medical Uses of Architecture." In *Buildings and Society: Essays on the Social Development of the Built Environment*, edited by Anthony D. King, 32–50. London: Routledge.

Foucault, Michel. 1978. *The History of Sexuality, Volume 1: An Introduction*. Translated by Robert Hurley. New York: Vintage Books.

Foucault, Michel. 1980. *Power/Knowledge: Selected Interviews & Other Writings*, edited by Colin Gordon. New York: Vintage.

Foucault, Michel. 1982. "Afterword: The Subject and Power." In *Michel Foucault: Beyond Structuralism and Hermeneutics*, edited by Hubert L. Dreyffus and Paul Rabinow. New York: Harvester Wheatsheaf.

Foucault, Michel. 1994. *The Birth of the Clinic: An Archeology of Medical Perception*. Translated by Alan Mark Sheridan Smith. New York: Vintage Books.

Foucault, Michel. 2003. *Psychiatric Power: Lectures at the Collège de France 1973–1974*. New York: Picador.

Foucault, Michel. 2006. *History of Madness*. Translated by Jonathan Murphy and Jean Khalfa. London: Routledge.

Foucault, Michel. 2007. *Security, Territory, Population: Lectures at the Collège de France 1977–1978*. New York: Palgrave Macmillan.

Foucault, Michel. 2008. *The Birth of Biopolitics: Lectures at the Collège de France 1978–1979*. New York: Palgrave Macmillan.

Foucault, Michel. 2010. *The Government of Self and Others: Lectures at the Collège de France 1982–1983*. New York: Palgrave Macmillan.

Foucault, Michel. 2011. *Courage of Truth: The Government of Self and Others. Lectures at the Collège de France 1983–1984*. Translated by Graham Burchell. New York: Palgrave.

Foucault, Michel. 2012. *On the Government of the Living: Lectures at the Collège de France 1979–1980 and Oedipal Knowledge*. New York: Picador.

Foucault, Michel. 2017. *Subjectivity and Truth: Lectures at the Collège de France 1980–1981*. Translated by Graham Burchell. New York: Palgrave.

Fox, Marie, and Mo Ray. 2019. "No Pets Allowed? Companion Animals, Older People and Residential Care". *Medical Humanities* 45 (2): 211–222.

Fox, Nick. 1999. *Beyond Health: Postmodernism and Embodiment*. London: Free Association Books.

Freud, Sigmund. 2010. *The Interpretation of Dreams: The Complete and Definitive Text*. Translated by James Strachey. New York: Basic Books.

Fry, Tony. 2011. *Design As Politics*. Oxford: Berg.

Galbally, Megan, Anne Sved-Williams, Donna Kristianopulos, Kristine Mercuri, Phillipa Brown, and Anne Buist. 2019. "Comparison of Public Mother–Baby Psychiatric Units in Australia: Similarities, Strengths and Recommendations." *Australasian Psychiatry* 27 (2): 112–116.

Garrett, Charlotte, Beth Turner, and Anja Wittkowski. 2018. "Psychological and Psychosocial Interventions for Improving the Mental Health of Women Admitted to Mother and Baby Units in the United Kingdom." *Women's Health Research* 2 (1): 29–41.

Gillespie, Rosemary. 2002. "Architecture and Power: A Family Planning Clinic As a Case Study." *Health and Place* 8 (3): 211–220.

Gillham, Rebecca, and Anja Wittkowski. 2015. "Outcomes for Women Admitted to a Mother and Baby Unit: A Systematic Review." *International Journal of Women's Health* 7: 459–476.

Glangeaud-Freudenthal, Nine M.-C., Anne Laure Sutter, Anne-Claire Thieulin, Véronique Dagens-Lafont, Marie-Agathe Zimmermann, Alain Debourg, B. Massari, Odile Cazas, Rafaële Cammas, Christine Rainelli, François Poinso, Michel Maron, Sylvie Nezelof, P.-Y. Ancel, and B. Khoshnood. 2011. "Inpatient Mother-and-Child Postpartum Psychiatric Care: Factors Associated with Improvement in Maternal Mental Health." *European Psychiatry* 26 (4): 215–223.

Glangeaud-Freudenthal, Nine M.-C., Anne-Laure Sutter-Dallay, Anne-Claire Thieulin, Véronique Dagens, Marie-Agathe Zimmermann, Alain Debourg, Corinne Amzallag, Odile Cazas, Rafaële Cammas, Marie-Emmanuelle Klopfert, Christine Rainelli, Pascale Tielemans, Claudine Mertens, Michel Maron, Sylvie Nezelof, and F. Poinso. 2013. "Predictors of Infant Foster Care in Cases of Maternal Psychiatric Disorders." *Social Psychiatry and Psychiatric Epidemiology* 48 (4): 553–561.

Glangeaud-Freudenthal, Nine M.-C., Christine Rainelli, Odile Cazas, Sylvie Nezelof, Michel Dugnat, François Poinso, and Anne-Laure Sutter-Dallay. 2016. "Inpatient Mother and Baby Psychiatric Units (MBUs) and Day Cares." In *Joint Care of Parents and Infants in Perinatal Psychiatry*, edited by Anne-Laure Sutter-Dallay, Nine M.-C. Glangeaud-Freudenthal, Antoine Guedeney, and Anita Riecher-Rössler, 147–164. Cham: Springer.

Glangeaud-Freudenthal, Nine M. C., Louise M. Howard, and Anne-Laure Sutter-Dallay. 2014. "Treatment – Mother-Infant Inpatient Units." *Best Practice & Research Clinical Obstetrics and Gynaecology* 28 (1): 147–157.

Glangeaud-Freudenthal, Nine M.-C., and The MBU-SMF Working Group. 2004. "Mother-Baby Psychiatric Units (MBUs): National Data Collection in France and in Belgium (1999–2000)." *Archives of Women's Mental Health* 7 (1): 59–64.

Golembiewski, Jan. 2010. "Start Making Sense: Applying a Salutogenic Model to Architectural Design for Psychiatric Care." *Facilities* 28 (3–4): 100–117.

Green, Debra J., Kristina Hofberg, Caroline Carr, Tina Fanneran, and Athula Sumathipala. 2016. "A 10-Year History of Perinatal Care at the Brockington Mother and Baby Unit Stafford." *Archives of Women's Mental Health* 19 (3): 507–513.

Gressier, Florence, Virginie Guillard, Odile Cazas, Bruno Falissard, Nine M.-C. Glangeaud-Freudenthal, and Anne-Laure Sutter-Dallay. 2017. "Risk Factors for Suicide Attempt in Pregnancy and the Post-Partum Period in Women with Serious Mental Illnesses." *Journal of Psychiatric Research* 84: 284–291.

Grosz, Elizabeth. 2005. *Time Travels: Feminism, Nature, Power*. Crows Nest: Allen & Unwin.

Grube, Michael. 2005. "Inpatient Treatment of Women with Postpartum Psychiatric Disorders – The Role of the Male Partners." *Archives of Women's Mental Health* 8 (3): 163–170.

Hafner, Diane. 2013. "Objects, Agency and Context: Australian Aboriginal Expressions of Connection in Relation to Museum Artefacts." *Journal of Material Culture* 18 (4): 347–366.

Hayward, Stephen. 1998. "'Good Design Is Largely a Matter of Common Sense': Questioning the Meaning and Ownership of Twentieth Century Orthodoxy." *The Journal of Design History* 11 (3): 217–233.

Hickman, Clare. 2009. "Cheerful Prospects and Tranquil Restoration: The Visual Experience of Landscape As Part of the Therapeutic Regime of the British Asylum, 1800–60." *History of Psychiatry* 20 (4): 425–441.

Hill, Rebecca, Daphne Law, Chris Yelland, and Anne Sved Williams. 2019. "Treatment of Postpartum Psychosis in a Mother-Baby Unit: Do Both Mother and Baby Benefit?" *Australasian Psychiatry* 27 (2): 121–124.

Hipwell, Alison E., Frits A. Goossens, Edward C. Melhuish, and Ratnesh Kumar. 2000. "Severe Maternal Psychopathology and Infant-Mother Attachment." *Development and Psychopathology* 12 (2): 157–175.

Howard, Louise, Nisha Shah, Margaret Salmon, and Louis Appleby. 2003. "Predictors of Social Services Supervision of Babies of Mothers with Mental Illness After Admission to a Psychiatric Mother and Baby Unit." *Social Psychiatry and Psychiatric Epidemiology* 38 (8): 450–455.

Howard, Louise M. 2000. "The Separation of Mothers and Babies in the Treatment of Postpartum Psychotic Disorders in Britain 1900–1960." *Archives of Women's Mental Health* 3 (1): 1–5.

Irigaray, Luce. 1991. *Marine Lover of Friedrich Nietzsche*. Translated by Gillian C. Gill. New York: Columbia University Press.

Johansson, Inger M., Ingela Skärsäter, and Ella Danielson. 2006. "The Health-Care Environment on a Locked Psychiatric Ward: An Ethnographic Study." *International Journal of Mental Health Nursing* 15 (4): 242–250.

Johansson, Inger M., Ingela Skärsäter, and Ella Danielson. 2007. "Encounters in a Locked Psychiatric Ward Environment." *Journal of Psychiatric and Mental Health Nursing* 14 (4): 366–372.

Kanyeredzi, Ava, Steven D. Brown, Laura McGrath, Paula Reavey, and Ian Tucker. 2019. "The Atmosphere of the Ward: Attunements and Attachments of Everyday Life for Patients on a Medium-Secure Forensic Psychiatric Unit." *The Sociological Review* 67 (2): 444–466.

Kaup, Migette L. 2011. "The Significance of the Door in Nursing Homes: A Symbol of Control in the Domestic Sphere." *Home Cultures* 8 (1): 25–41.

Keller, Heidi. 2016. "Attachment. A Pancultural Need but a Cultural Construct." *Current Opinion in Psychology* 8: 59–63.

Kelly, Maura. 2016. "Sex Versus Gender Categorization." In *The Wiley Blackwell Encyclopedia of Gender and Sexuality Studie*s, edited by Nancy Naples, Maithree Wickramasinghe, and Angela Wong Wai Ching. Malden, Massachusetts: Wiley Blackwell.

Kemp, Natalie. 2011. "Fathers' Experiences of a Mother and Baby Unit: A Qualitative Study." Doctor of Clinical Psychology diss., Canterbury Christ Church University.

Kennedy, Jennifer, and Tracy Fortune. 2014. "Women's Experiences of Being in an Acute Psychiatric Unit: An Occupational Perspective." *British Journal of Occupational Therapy* 77 (6): 296–303.

Kenny, Maeve, Susan Conroy, Carmine M. Pariante, Gertrude Seneviratne, and Susan Pawlby. 2013. "Mother-Infant Interaction in Mother and Baby Unit Patients: Before and After Treatment." *Journal of Psychiatric Research* 47 (9): 1192–1198.

Korteland, Tim W., Kathelijne M. Koorengevel, Irina E. Poslawsky, and Berno van Meijel. 2019. "Nursing Interventions for Patients with Postpartum Psychosis Hospitalized in a Psychiatric Mother–Baby Unit: A Qualitative Study." *Journal of Psychiatric and Mental Health Nursing* 26 (7–8): 254–264.

Lacan, Jacques. 2006. *Écrits*. Translated by Bruce Fink. New York: Norton.

Laing, Ronald David. 1967. *The Politics of Experience.* New York: Pantheon.

Le Treut, Laure, François Poinso, Pauline Grandgeorge, Elisabeth Jouve, Michel Dugnat, Joshua Sparrow, and Jokthan Guivarch. 2018. "Infant Psychomotor Development in Cases of Maternal Postpartum Depression: Observation of a Mother and Baby Unit." *Mental Illness* 10 (1): 27–30.

Leach, Andrew, William M. Taylor, and Lee Stickells. 2013. "Architecture, Evidence, and 'Evidentiality'." *Architectural Theory Review* 18 (1): 1–7.

Lemke, Thomas. 2015. "New Materialisms: Foucault and the Government of Things." *Theory Culture and Society* 27 (1): 130–152.

Long, Clive G., Vikki Langford, Rebecca Clay, Lorraine Craig, and Clive R. Hollin. 2011. "Architectural Change and the Effects on the Perceptions of the Ward Environment in a Medium Secure Unit for Women." *The British Journal of Forensic Practice* 13 (3): 205–212.

Main, T. F. 1958. "Mothers with Children in a Psychiatric Hospital." *The Lancet* 272 (7051): 845–847.

Maizel, S., S. Kandel Katzenelson, and V. Fainstein. 2005. "The Jerusalem Psychiatric Mother-Baby Unit." *Archives of Women's Mental Health* 8 (3): 200–202.

Marrs, Jennifer, Jill Cossar, and Anna Wroblewska. 2014. "Keeping the Family Together and Bonding: A Father's Role in a Perinatal Mental Health Unit." *Journal of Reproductive and Infant Psychology* 32 (4): 340–354.

Martin, Daryl, Sarah Nettleton, Christina Buse, Lindsay Prior, and Julia Twigg. 2015. "Architecture and Health Care: A Place for Sociology." *Sociology of Health & Illness* 37 (7): 1007–1022.

Marzano, Marco. 2007. "Informed Consent, Deception, and Research Freedom in Qualitative Research." *Qualitative Inquiry* 13 (3): 417–436.

Masciantonio, Sonia. 2015. "Mothering & Mental Illness: An Ethnography of Attachment in an Institutional Context." PhD diss., University of Adelaide.

Massey, Doreen. 1994. *Space, Place and Gender.* Minneapolis: University of Minnesota Press.

McCarthy, Christine. 2005. "Towards a Definition of Interiority." *Space and Culture* 8 (2): 112–125.

McClintock, Anne. 1995. *Imperial Leather: Race: Gender and Sexuality in the Colonial Context.* New York: Routledge.

McLaughlan, Rebecca. 2017. "Learning from Evidence-Based Medicine: Exclusions and Opportunities within Health Care Environments Research." *Design for Health* 1 (2): 210–228.

Meacham, Standish. 1999. *Regaining Paradise: Englishness and the Early Garden City Movement.* New Haven: Yale University Press.

Meltzer-Brody, Samantha, Anna R. Brandon, Brenda Pearson, Lynne Burns, Christena Raines, Elizabeth Bullard, and David Rubinow. 2014. "Evaluating the Clinical Effectiveness of a Specialized Perinatal Psychiatry Inpatient Unit." *Archives of Women's Mental Health* 17 (2): 107–113.

Miller, Daniel. 2001. "Possessions." In *Home Possessions*, edited by Daniel Miller, 107–121. Oxford: Berg.

Montgomery-Downs, Hawley, Robyn Stremler, and Salvatore P. Insana. (2013). "Postpartum Sleep in New Mothers and Fathers." *The Open Sleep Journal* 6 (1): 87–97.

Nair, Revi, Justin Bilszta, Nilam Salam, Nadia Shafira, and Anne Buist. 2010. "Client Evaluation of a Specialist Inpatient Parent-Infant Psychiatric Service." *Australasian Psychiatry* 18 (6): 573–578.

National Institute for Health and Care Excellence. 2014. *Antenatal and Postnatal Mental Health: Clinical Management and Service Guidance.* London: NICE.

Neil, S., H. Sanderson, and Angelika Wieck. 2006. "A Satisfaction Survey of Women Admitted to a Psychiatric Mother and Baby Unit in the Northwest of England." *Archives of Women's Mental Health* 9 (2): 109–112.

Noorlander, Y., Veerle Bergink, and Mijke P. van den Berg. 2008. "Perceived and Observed Mother–Child Interaction at Time of Hospitalization and Release in Postpartum Depression and Psychosis." *Archives of Women's Mental Health* 11 (1): 49–56.

Novotná, Gabriela, Karen Urbanoski, and Brian Rush. 2011. "Client-Centred Design of Residential Addiction and Mental Health Care Facilities: Staff Perceptions of their Work Environment." *Qualitative Health Research* 21 (11): 1527–1538.

Oakley, Ann. 1974. *Housewife.* London: Allen Lane.

O'Mahony, Joyce Maureen, Tam Truong Donnelly, Shelly Raffin Bouchal, and David Este. 2013. "Cultural Background and Socioeconomic Influence of Immigrant and Refugee Women Coping with Postpartum Depression." *Journal of Immigrant and Minority Health* 15 (2): 300–314.

Pearce, Linda. 2018. "Translating Across Disciplines: On Coding Interior Architecture Theory to Advance Complex Indoor Environment Quality." *Buildings* 8 (7): 82–101.

Pevsner, Niklaus. 1975. *Pioneers of Modern Design: From William Morris to Walter Gropius*. Harmondsworth: Pelican.

Plato. 1935. *The Republic of Plato*. Translated by John Llewelyn Davies and David James Vaughan. London: Macmillan.

Poinso, François, M. P. Gay, Nine M. C. Glangeaud-Freudenthal, and Marcel Rufo. 2002. "Care in a Mother-Baby Psychiatric Unit: Analysis of Separation at Discharge." *Archives of Women's Mental Health* 5 (2): 49–58.

Redhouse, Nicola. 2019. *Unlike the Heart: A Memoir of Brain and Mind.* St. Lucia: University of Queensland Press.

Reid, Holly, Angelika Wieck, Andrew Matrunola, and Anja Wittkowski. (2017). "The Experiences of Fathers When Their Partners Are Admitted with Their Infants to a Psychiatric Mother and Baby Unit." *Clinical Psychology & Psychotherapy* 24 (4): 919–931.

Reilly, Nicole, Gemma Turner, Jamilie Taouk, and Marie-Paule Austin. 2019. "'Singing with Your Baby': An Evaluation of Group Singing Sessions for Women Admitted to a Specialist Mother-Baby Unit." *Archives of Women's Mental Health* 22 (1): 123–127.

Rendell, Jane. 2000. "Introduction: Gender, Space, Architecture." In *Gender Space and Architecture: An interdisciplinary introduction*, edited by Jane Rendell, Barbara Penner, and Iain Borden, 225–239. London: Routledge.

Riggs, Damien, Clare Bartholomaeus, Clemence Due, and Kathleen Connellan. 2020. "Love and Motherhood in Louis Theroux's Mothers on the Edge." *Feminist Media Studies* 20 (4): 590–593.

Rose, Nicholas. 1998. *Inventing Ourselves: Psychology, Power and Personhood.* Cambridge: Cambridge University Press.

Rose, Nicholas. 1999. *Governing the Soul: The Shaping of the Private Self.* London: Free Association Books.

Roser, Max, and Hannah Ritchie. 2019. "Maternal Mortality." *OurWorldInData.org*. https://ourworldindata.org/maternal-mortality'

Royal Australian & New Zealand College of Psychiatrists. 2015. *Position Statement 57: Mothers, Babies and Psychiatric Inpatient Treatment*. RANZCP. https://www.ranzcp.org/home

Salmon, Margaret, Kathryn Abel, Lis Cordingley, Trevor Friedman, and Louis Appleby. 2003. "Clinical and Parenting Skills Outcomes Following Joint Mother–Baby Psychiatric Admission." *Australian and New Zealand Journal of Psychiatry* 37 (5): 556–562.

Savage, Jan. 2000. "Ethnography and Health Care." *British Medical Journal* 321: 1400–1402.

Scott, Joan Wallach. 2000. "Excerpts from Gender: A Useful Category in Historical Analysis." In *Gender Space and Architecture: An Interdisciplinary Introduction*, edited by Jane Rendell, Barbara Penner and Iain Borden, 74–87. London: Routledge.

Seneviratne, Gertrude, Susan Conroy, and Maureen Marks. 2003. "Parenting Assessment in a Psychiatric Mother and Baby Unit." *The British Journal of Social Work* 33 (4): 535–555.

Shaftoe, Henry. 2012. *Convivial Urban Spaces: Creating Effective Public Places.* London: Routledge.

Shepley, Mardelle McCuskey, Angela Watson, Francis Pitts, Anne Garrity, Elizabeth Spelman, Andrea Fronsman, and Janhawi Kelkar. 2017. "Mental and Behavioural Health Settings: Importance and Effectiveness of Environmental Qualities and Features As Perceived by Staff." *Journal of Environmental Psychology* 50: 37–50.

Sinding, Christina. 2010. "Using Institutional Ethnography to Understand the Production of Healthcare Disparities." *Qualitative Health Research* 20 (12): 1656–1633.

Skeggs, Beverley, and Helen Wood. 2011. "Turning It On Is a Class Act: Immediated Object Relations with Television." *Media, Culture & Society* 33 (6): 941–951.

Sparke, Penny. 2008. "Perspective: The Modern Interior Revisited." *Journal of Interior Design* 34 (1): v–xii.

Stephenson, Lucy A., Alastair J. D. Macdonald, Gertrude Seneviratne, Freddie Waites, and Susan Pawlby. 2018. "Mother and Baby Units Matter: Improved Outcomes for Both." *BJPsych Open* 4: 119–125.

Stichler, Jaynelle F. 2008. "Healing by Design." *Health Facility Design* 38 (12): 505–509.

Sutter-Dallay, Anne-Laure, and Nicole Guedeney. 2016. "Introduction: History." In *Joint Care of Parents and Infants in Perinatal Psychiatry*, edited by Anne-Laure Sutter-Dallay, Nine M.-C. Glangeaud-Freudenthal, Antoine Guedeney, and Anita Riecher-Rössler, 3–11. Cham: Springer.

Tasca, Cecelia, Mariangela Rapetti, Maura Giovanni Carta, and Bianca Fadda. 2012. "Women and Hysteria in the History of Mental Health." *Clinical Practice & Epidemiology in Mental Health* 8: 110–119.

Theroux, Louis, dir. 2019. *Louis Theroux: Mothers on the Edge*. BBC 2 Productions.

Torgrimson, Britta N., and Christopher T. Minson. 2005. "Sex and Gender: What Is the Difference?" *Journal of Applied Physiology* 99: 785–787.

Tucker, Ian M., Steven D. Brown, Ava Kanyeredzi, Laura McGrath, and Paula Reavey. 2019. "Living 'In Between' Outside and Inside: The Forensic Psychiatric Unit As Impermanent Assemblage." *Health and Place* 55: 29–36.

Turner, Beth, Charlotte Garrett, and Anja Wittkowski. 2018. "Male Partners of Women Admitted to Mother and Baby Units in the United Kingdom: A Survey of Available Psychosocial and Psychological Interventions." *Women's Health Research* 1 (1): 25–36.

Ulrich, Roger, Craig Zimring, Xuemei Zhu, Jennifer DuBose, Hyun-Bo Seo, Young-Seon Choi, Xiaobo Quan, and Anjali Joseph. 2008. "A Review of the Research Literature on Evidence-Based Healthcare Design." *Health Environments Research & Design Journal* 1 (3): 101–165.

Urbanoski, Karen. 2013. "Does the Redesign of a Psychiatric Inpatient Unit Change the Treatment Process and Outcomes?" *Psychiatric Services* 64 (8): 804–807.

Van Puyvelde, Martine, Helena Rodrigues, Gerrit Loots, Lotta De Coster, Kevin Du Ville, Liesbeth Matthijs, David Simcock, and Nathalie Pattyn. 2014. "Shall We Dance? Music As a Port of Entrance to Maternal-Infant Intersubjectivity in a Context of Postnatal Depression." *Infant Mental Health Journal* 35 (3): 220–232.

Vliegen, Nicole, Patrick Luyten, Avi Besser, Sara Casalin, Stefan Kempke, and Eileen Tang. 2010. "Stability and Change in Levels of Depression and Personality:

A Follow-Up Study of Postpartum Depressed Mothers That Were Hospitalized in a Mother-Infant Unit." *The Journal of Nervous and Mental Disease* 198 (1): 45–51.

Vliegen, Nicole, Sara Casalin, Patrick Luyten, Ria Docx, Marijs Lenaerts, Eileen Tang, and Stefan Kempke. 2013. "Hospitalization-Based Treatment for Postpartum Depressed Mothers and Their Babies: Rationale, Principles, and Preliminary Follow-Up Data." *Psychiatry* 76 (2): 150–168.

Wagstaff, Adam. 2000. "Socioeconomic Inequalities in Child Mortality: Comparisons Across Nine Developing Countries." *Bulletin of the World Health Organization* 78 (1): 19–29.

Walker, Lynne. 2000. "Women and Architecture." In *Gender, Space, Architecture: An Interdisciplinary Introduction*, edited by Jane Rendell, Barbara Penner, and Iain Borden, 244–257. London: Routledge.

Wan, Ming Wai, Alison L. Warburton, Louis Appleby, and Kathryn M. Abel. 2007. "Mother and Baby Unit Admissions: Feasibility Study Examining Child Outcomes 4–6 Years On." *Australian and New Zealand Journal of Psychiatry* 41 (2): 150–156.

White, Robert D. 2011. "The Newborn Intensive Care Unit Environment of Care: How We Got Here, Where We're Headed, and Why." *Seminars in Perinatology* 35 (1): 2–7.

Winnicott, Donald W. 1953. "Transitional Objects and Transitional Phenomena – A Study of the First Not-Me Possession." *International Journal of Psycho-Analysis* 34: 89–97.

Wittkowski, Anja, Dougal J. Hare, and Rebecca Gillham. 2019. "Using the Repertory Grid Technique to Explore the Experience of Compassion by Mothers in a Mother and Baby Unit." *Midwifery* 75: 24–32.

Wood, Victoria, Sarah E. Curtis, Wil Gesler, Ian H. Spencer, Helen J. Close, James Mason, and Joe G. Reilly. 2013. "Creating 'Therapeutic Landscapes' for Mental Health Carers in Inpatient Settings: A Dynamic Perspective on Permeability and Inclusivity." *Social Science & Medicine* 91: 122–129.

Wood, Victoria J., Wil Gesler, Sarah E. Curtis, Ian H. Spencer, Helen J. Close, James Mason, and Joe G. Reilly. 2015. "'Therapeutic Landscapes' and the Importance of Nostalgia, Solastalgia, Salvage and Abandonment for Psychiatric Hospital Design." *Health & Place* 33: 83–89.

Wright, Tanya, Suzanne Stevens, and Trecia A. Wouldes. 2018. "Mothers and Their Infants Co-Admitted to a Newly Developed Mother-Baby Unit: Characteristics and Outcomes." *Infant Mental Health Journal* 39 (6): 707–717.

Wright, Tanya, Tanisha Jowsey, Josephine Stanton, Hinemoa Elder, Suzanne Stevens, and Trecia A. Wouldes. 2018. "Patient Experience of a Psychiatric Mother Baby Unit." *PLoS One* 13 (5): e0198241.

Yelland, Chris, Teresa Girke, Charlotte Tottman, and Anne Sved Williams. 2015. "Clinical Characteristics and Mental Health Outcomes for Women Admitted to an Australian Mother–Baby Unit: A Focus on Borderline Personality Disorder and Emotional Dysregulation?" *Australasian Psychiatry* 23 (6): 683–687.

Index

Page references for figures are italicized

About the Authors

Clare Bartholomaeus is a research fellow in the Melbourne Graduate School of Education at the University of Melbourne and an adjunct research fellow in the College of Education, Psychology and Social Work, Flinders University. She is the author or coauthor of over fifty publications in the areas of gender studies, education, health, and family studies, including *Transgender People and Education* (with Damien Riggs, Palgrave Macmillan, 2017).

Kathleen Connellan is a creative therapist, retired from thirty years of university teaching and research in art, architecture, and design. She has published widely across all these fields including specific studies into the meaning of home, and most recently, the healing effects of art: *Dreaming, Healing and Imaginative Arts Practice* (Routledge, 2019).

Clemence Due is a senior lecturer in psychology at The University of Adelaide. Her research expertise lies in the areas of mental health and well-being for families, including culturally and linguistically diverse peoples, as well as grief following pregnancy or neonatal loss. Her research is typically applied, and she works closely with communities to ensure that it meets their needs and leads to changes in policy and practice.

Damien W. Riggs is a professor in psychology at Flinders University and an Australian Research Council Future Fellow. He is the author of over 200 publications in the areas of gender, family, and mental health, including *Diverse Pathways to Parenthood: From Narratives to Practice* (Academic Press, 2019).

www.ingramcontent.com/pod-product-compliance
Ingram Content Group UK Ltd.
Pitfield, Milton Keynes, MK11 3LW, UK
UKHW020842290926
15470UKWH00004B/1494

9 781498 592918